This book is dedicated to those men and women who have advanced the frontiers of medical knowledge.

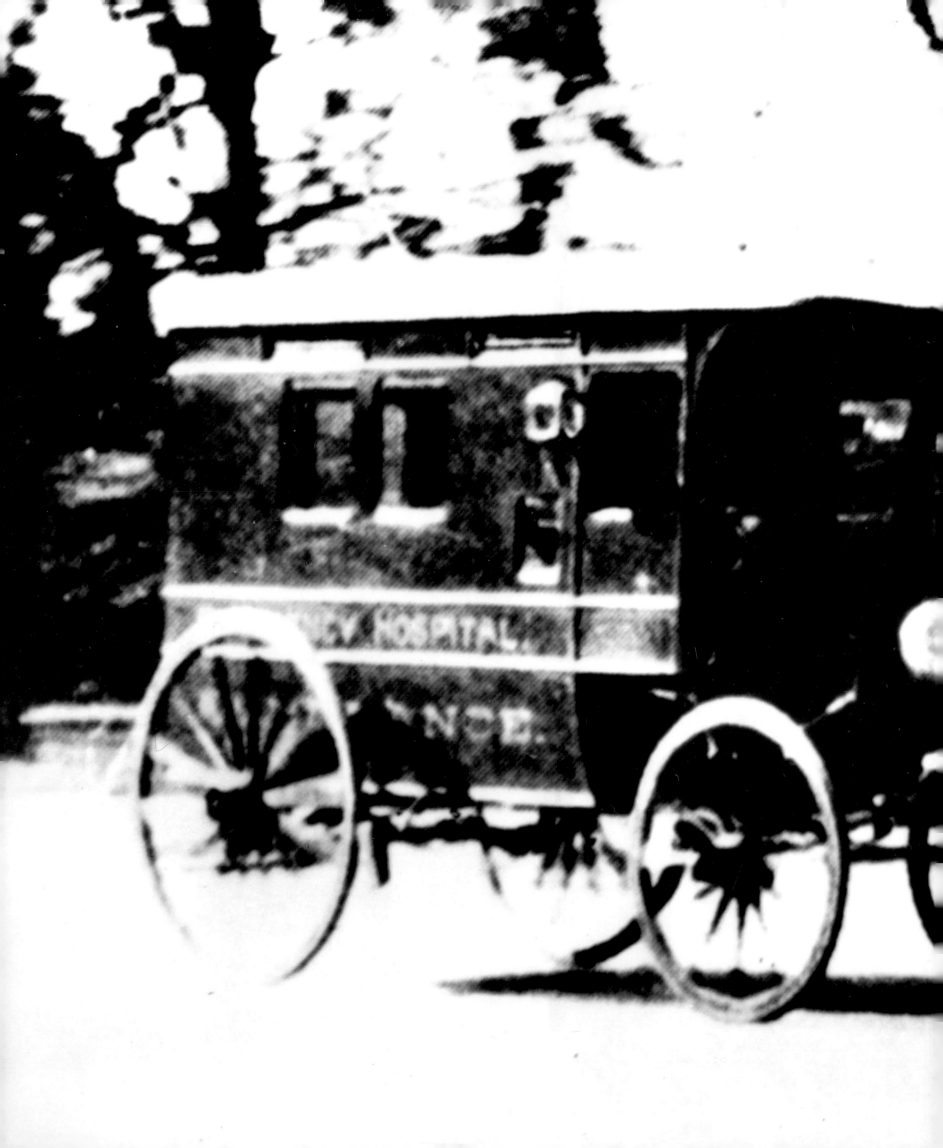

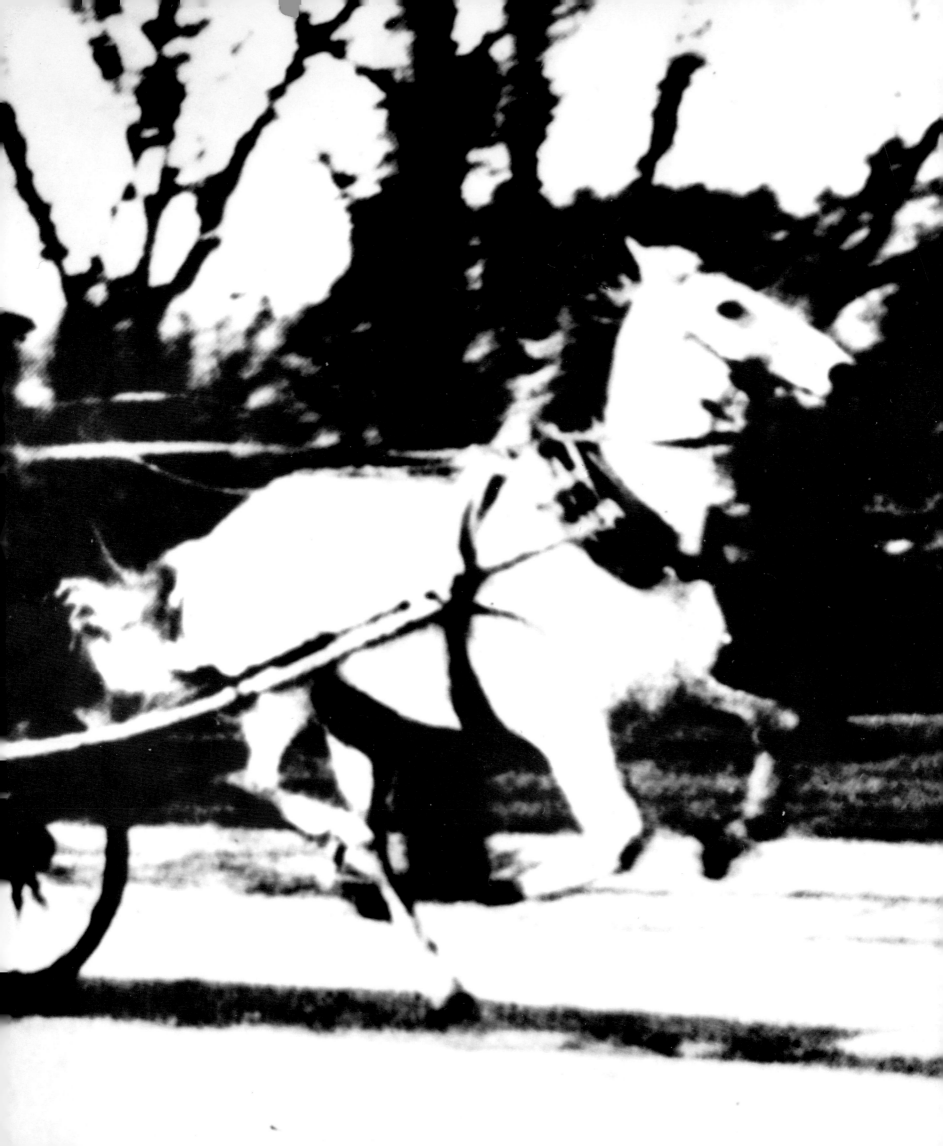

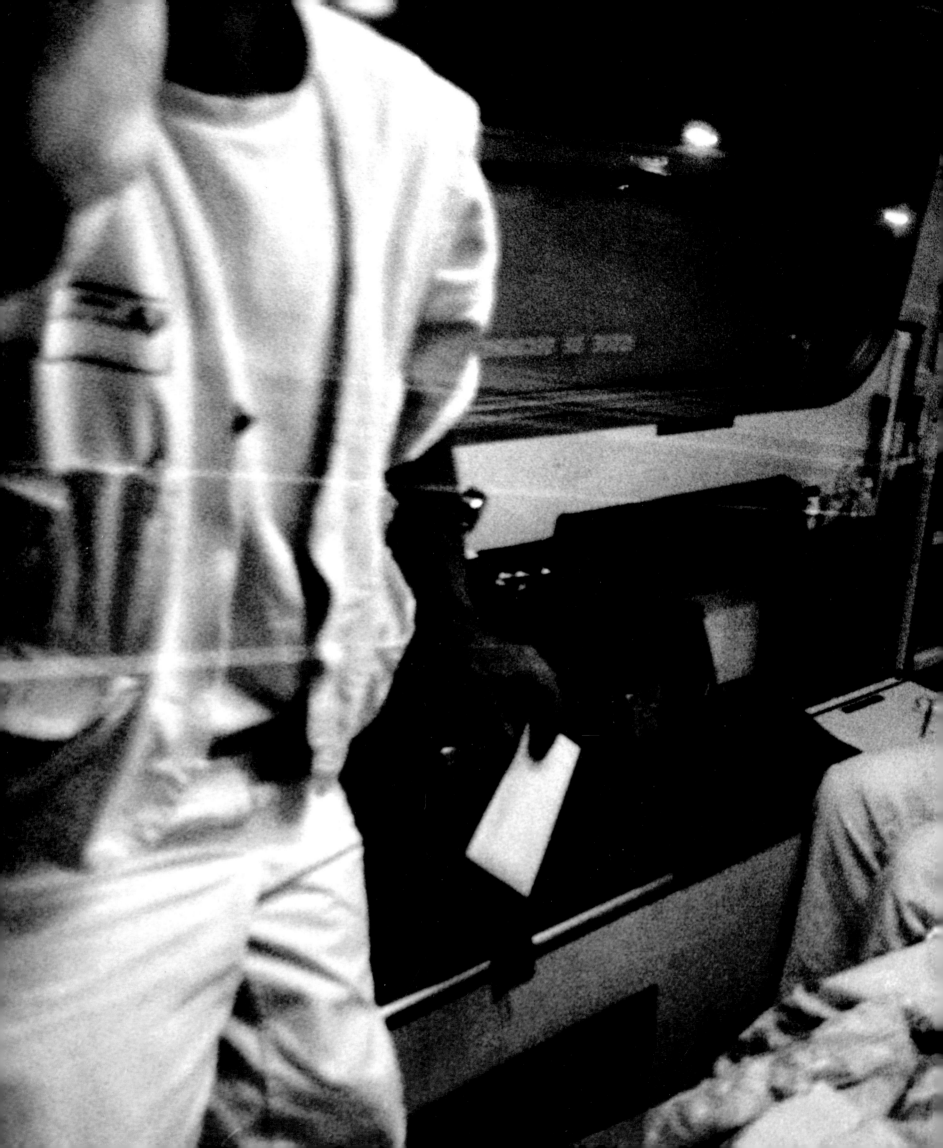

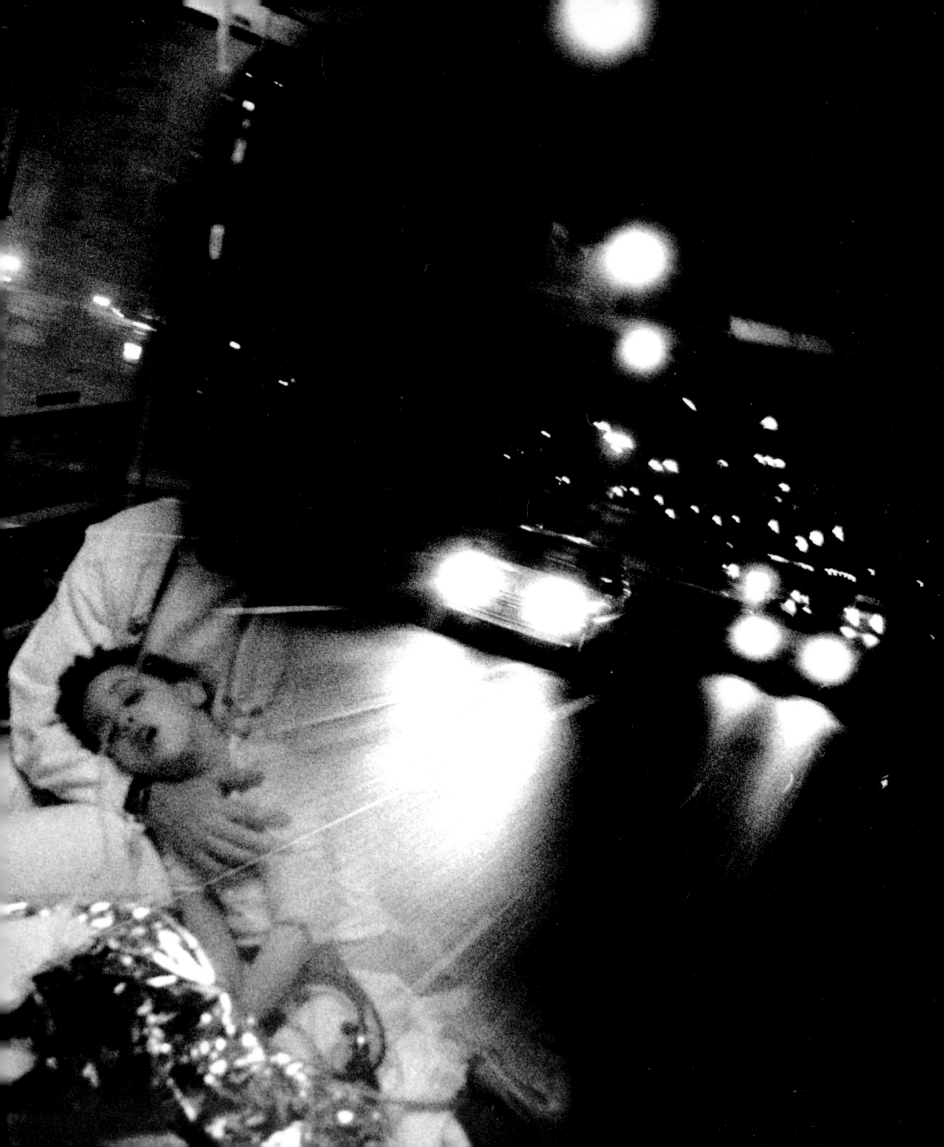

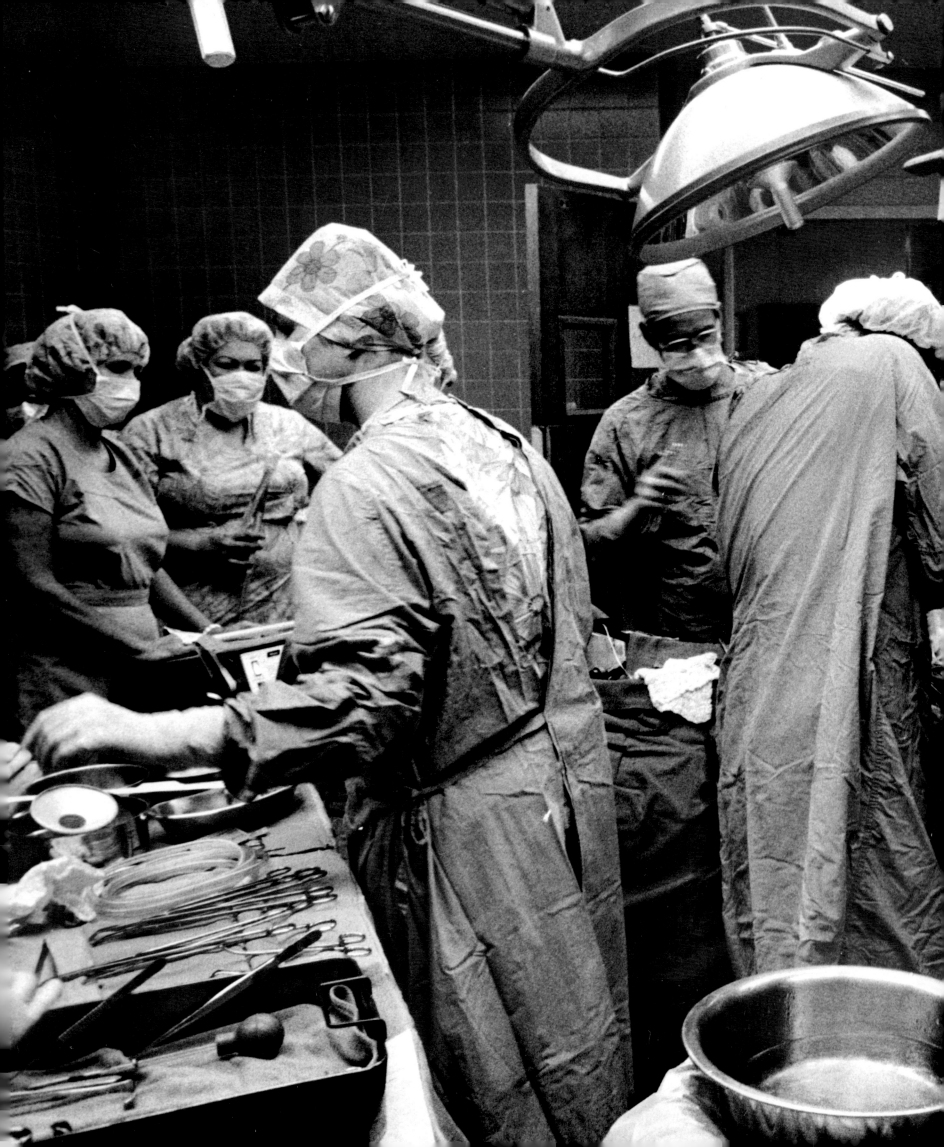

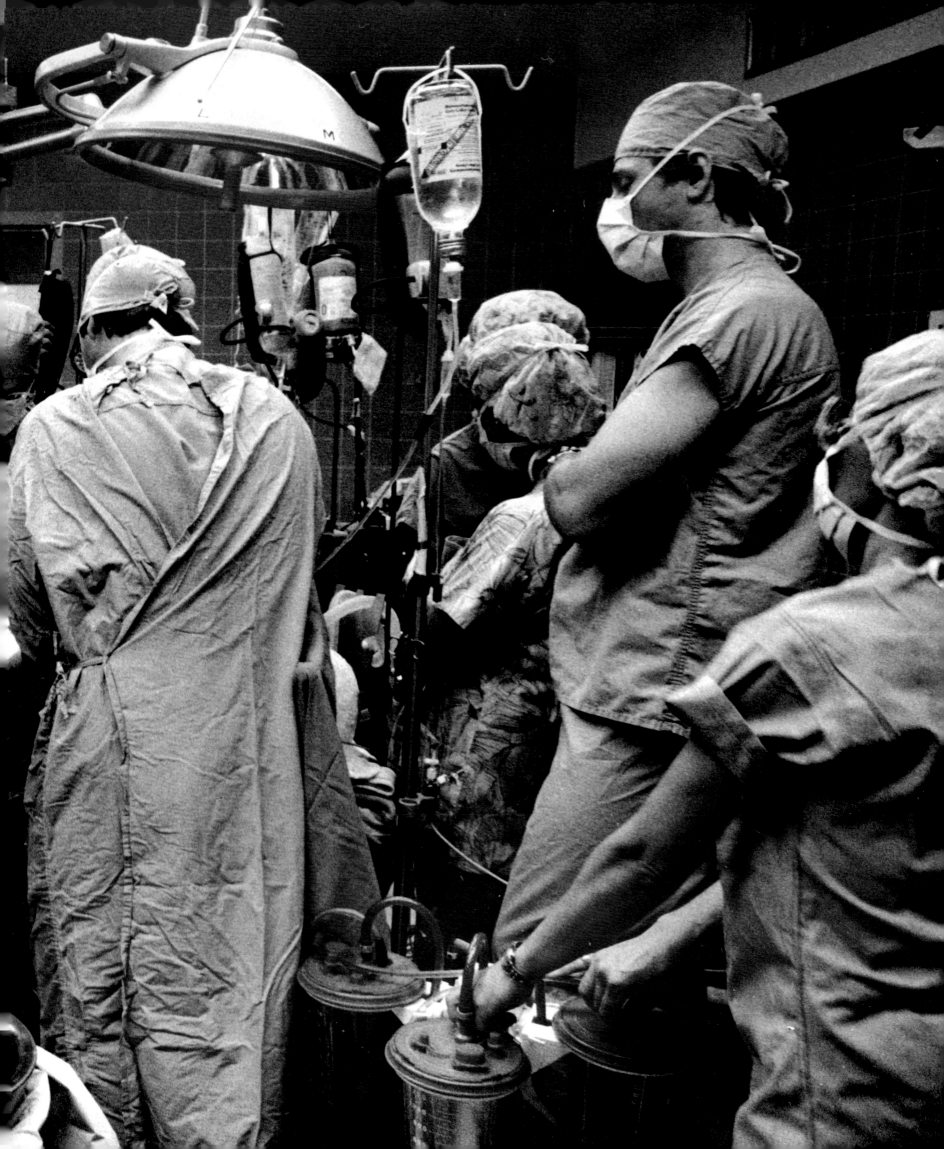

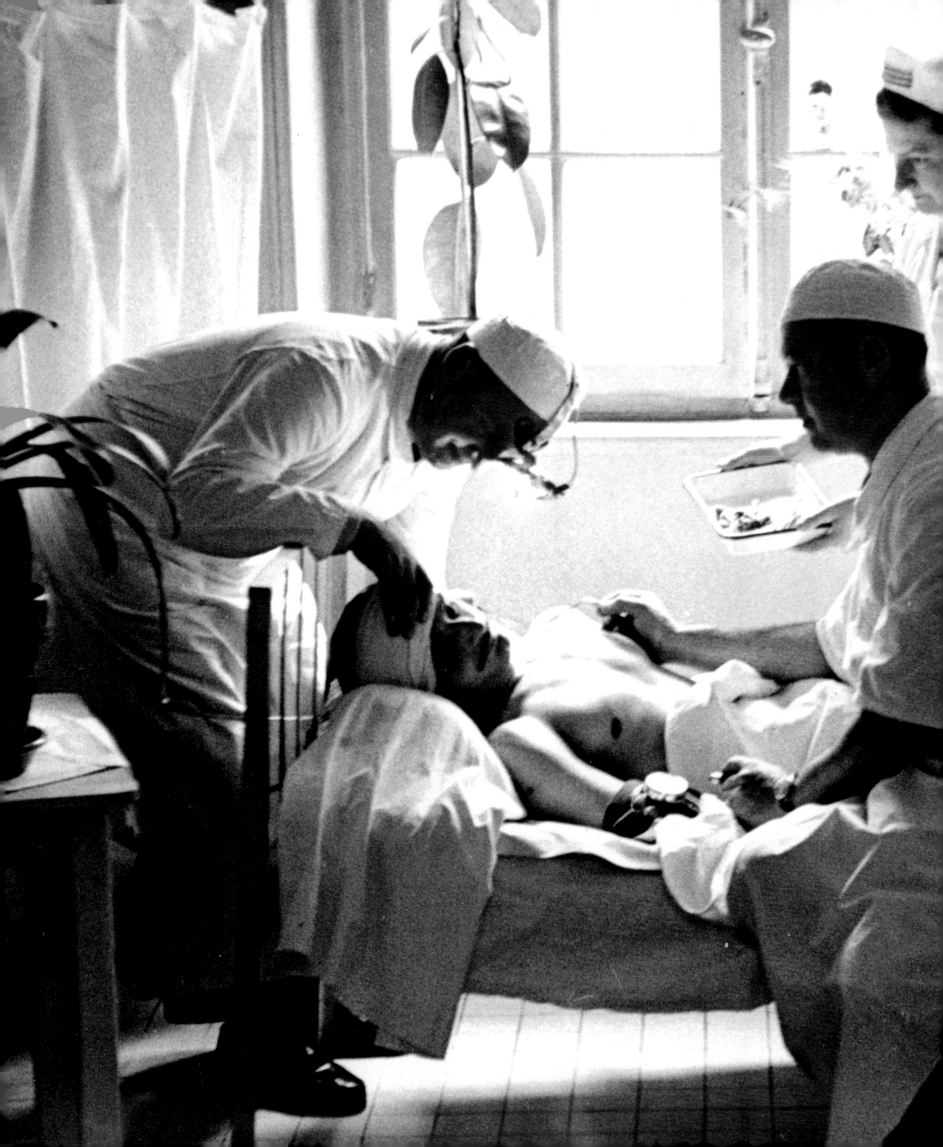

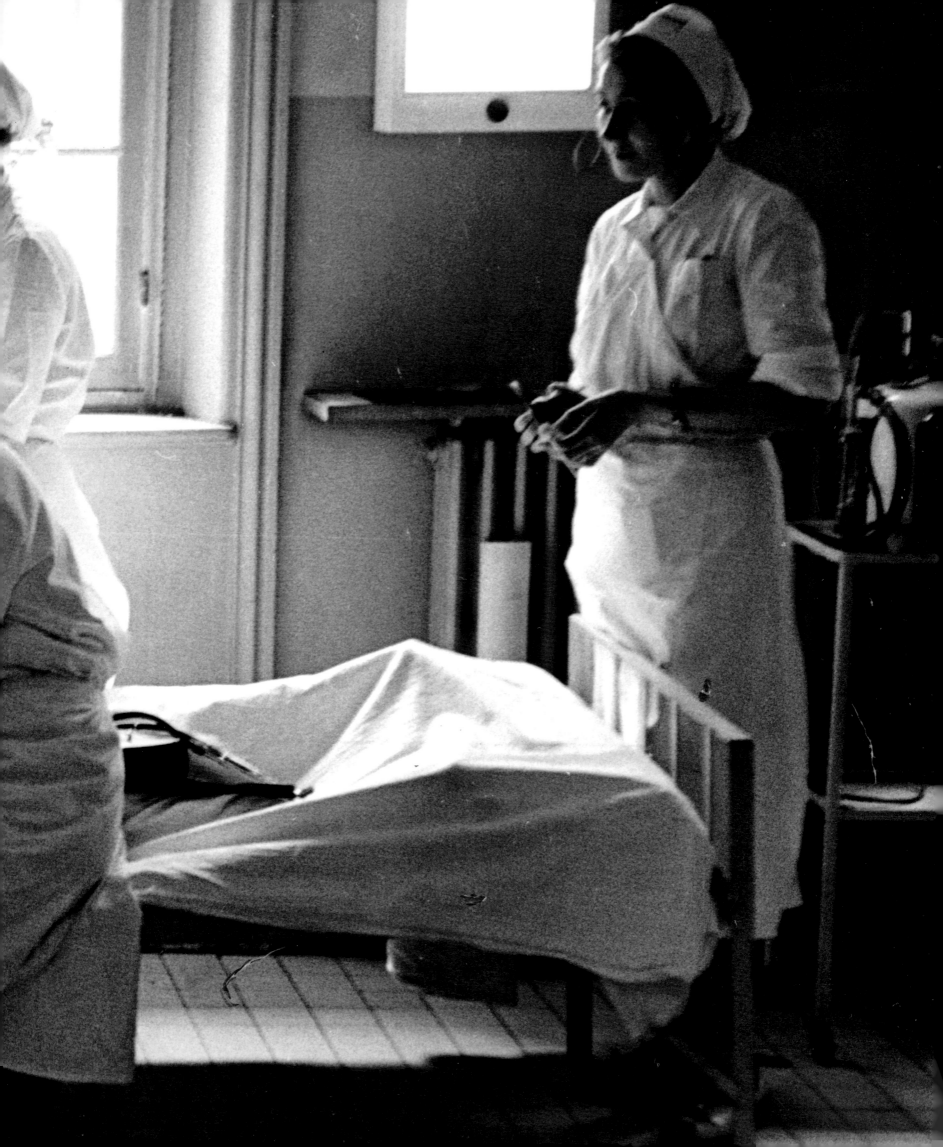

The companies below generously helped to provide the necessary funding and support to tell the story of medicine's great journey.

OLYMPUS

HEALTH Magazine

 Light Source Computer Imaging, Inc.

Eastman Kodak Company

MEDICINE'S GREAT JOURNEY

JOURNEY

One Hundred Years of Healing

Created by Rick Smolan and Phillip Moffitt

Introduction by Dr. Robert Coles
Text by Richard Flaste

Edited by Nan Richardson, Catherine Chermayeff, and Thomas K. Walker

Produced by Callaway Editions

A Bulfinch Press Book
Little, Brown and Company
Boston • Toronto • London

Jacket front: 1948. The Country Doctor. Photographed by W. E. Smith (detail; image in full on page 104).

Jacket back: Circa 1847. The doctor with his bag. Photographed by L. C. Dillon.

Pages ii-iii: Circa 1890-1900. Horsedrawn ambulance. Rush-Presbyterian-St. Luke's Medical Center Archives, Chicago.

Page iv-v: 1991. The SAMU (Service d'Aide Médicale Urgente), emergency ambulance service in Paris. Photographed by Luc Choquer.

Page vi-vii: 1964. Organ procurement procedure. Rush-Presbyterian-St. Luke's Medical Center Archives, Chicago. Photographed by David Joel.

Page viii-ix: Circa 1950s. Nurses and interns in the Fondation Rothschild, Paris, caring for their patient. Photographed by Edouard Boubat.

Medicine's Great Journey copyright © 1992 by Callaway Editions, Inc., and Mentor Capital, Inc.
Introduction copyright © 1992 by Robert Coles
Essay copyright © 1992 by Richard Flaste
Photographs copyrighted © 1992 in the names of the individual photographers or agencies
First Edition

ISBN 0-8212-1987-1
Library of Congress Catalog Card Number 92-54254

Edited by Nan Richardson and Catherine Chermayeff, Umbra Editions, Inc.
Designed by Thomas K. Walker, GRAF/x

Bulfinch Press is an imprint and trademark of Little, Brown and Company (Inc.)
Published simultaneously in Canada by Little, Brown & Company (Canada) Limited

PRINTED IN THE U.S.A.

Contents

Preface

As the twentieth century draws to a close, medical care has emerged as a critical issue for nations everywhere. Every day, news of yet another breakthrough in medical science appears, as medical researchers unravel another piece of the genetic code or lasers remove brain tumors without cutting into the skull. In every decade of this century, lifesaving advances from science and technology (which an earlier generation would have deemed miracles) have been perfected, incorporated into practice, and made widely available. This rapid and relentless march of progress is one of humanity's great triumphs. Unfortunately, at the same time, the exploding cost of good health care and its lack of availability for many people are issues of political debate whose outcome is of profound consequence to millions.

What is so often forgotten in the debate about medicine and health care is how incredibly young medical science is when compared to most of humanity's accomplishments. Civilization itself is at least nine thousand years old; democracy, as defined by the Greek city-state, is at least twenty-five hundred years old. Even the Industrial Revolution occurred over two hundred fifty years ago. Yet modern, scientific medicine is barely a century old. It is astounding how quickly we adjust the benchmark of what constitutes "good routine medical care." Drugs, tools, and procedures that are genuinely breathtaking in their very existence are quickly taken for granted.

One evening, my colleague, Rick Smolan, and I were discussing this phenomenon. It seemed to us that an important perspective is lost every time we, as a culture, lose a part of our "history"—in this instance, the rapid advancements in medicine. Rick suggested a powerful way to dramatize the scale of medicine's progress: through the use of photographs, letting readers see for themselves how quickly changes have occurred. Intriguingly, both photography and modern medicine emerged in the last century and the development of the two has been closely parallel. In fact, in the last decade, "imaging" has become one of the key tools of medicine. Rick and I were excited about the idea of creating a major, historical photographic record of modern medicine. We joined forces with a team of editors, writers, and researchers who initiated a worldwide archive search, which ultimately involved some six hundred photography collections in ten countries.

The result is *Medicine's Great Journey,* a fascinating book both for the medical story it tells as well as for the evolution of photography it reveals. These photographs present images of medical practices only a generation or two old; what may seem crude or simple to modern eyes were often critical steps on medicine's great journey of progress. These photographs also tell the story of the courage, inventiveness, and perseverance of the many doctors, nurses, and researchers who have made our lives immeasurably better.

Yet despite the progress in improving our health and life expectancy, we remain engaged in as ferocious a fight as ever against many *unnecessary* causes of disease and death— poverty, ignorance, malnutrition, and flagrant irresponsibility on the part of individuals in terms of their own health and by governments in their social and environmental policies. Be it infant mortality or cancer, we remain our own worst enemies, for it is human behavior that is most detrimental to human health, not viruses or bacteria.

It is our hope that this marvelous collection of photographs can help re-sensitize us to the miracles we have accomplished in health care and can help inspire a new determination in social policy and education that will lead us toward even greater accomplishments.

—*Phillip Moffitt*

The Past Is the Ground on Which We Walk

I will never forget the sight of one particular ward in the Massachusetts General Hospital in 1955, when a polio epidemic, the last before the Salk vaccine came into use, spread through metropolitan Boston. I was a medical resident then, spending long hours with patients who had "bulbar polio." The ward that day was filled with row upon row of metal cylinders filled with people, their heads visible at one end. These were iron lungs, breathing for those housed inside whose own breathing center in the brain-stem was inactivated by the polio virus. It was a heart-stopping sight.

One day, I went to visit an older physician whom I much admired. Indeed, I had written my college thesis on a long poem he'd written, for he was the legendary writing doctor—the poet William Carlos Williams. He was retired by then, and ailing, but his mind was still wonderfully shrewd, and visually alive. He was an amateur painter, and he loved to evoke the sight of things through words and images. As I described to him what I was seeing in that ward, his eyes widened and his face became animated. "Take a picture or two," he urged, "it will all pass, it will all be gone by the time you're my age."

At first I wasn't quite sure what he meant, but then I realized I was talking with an elderly physician whose medical memories had gradually lost their connection to the world's objective reality—erasures of progress. Dr. Williams, in fact, had already shared some of those memories with me: signs posted to warn people that someone inside a house had diphtheria, or public warnings issued about tuberculosis or syphilis. The photographs in this book bring all of that back—recollections Dr. Williams had conveyed to me, and moments in my own life. But I now understand that the old New Jersey doctor had something else in mind when he urged me to "take a picture or two." "The past matters more than we realize," he once said, explaining: "We walk on its ground, and if we don't know the soil, we're lost." He was always rendering images of that soil in his poems, his stories, his novels; and I know how eagerly he took to photographs, which in their own silent yet searching ways covered the same territory his verbal explorations meant to survey.

He had spent his life trying not only to envision the world, but to understand its assumptions, its aspirations and apprehensions. From this effort to understand came his famous clarion call, repeated again and again in his majestic, lyrical *Paterson:* "no ideas but in things." Williams' earthy, concrete mind feared big-shot, overwrought theories and generalizations, especially when they were used to replace a close look at life's everyday particulars, including those of history.

What follows in this book is a visual record of medicine's journey, the soil on which today's medicine walks. It is part of the territory he knew out of experience, or had heard described by his predecessors and teachers, for he graduated from the University of Pennsylvania Medical School at the very start of the twentieth century. As the book's photographs of early medicine reveal, in those days doctors lacked the wonderful cures we now can take for granted: antibiotics, cortisone, chemotherapy, and the radiological mastery we now possess through CAT scanning and MRI techniques. But as Dr. Williams often reminded me, there was no small amount of dignity and personal authority to be found among physicians: "We had our stethoscopes, and our microscopes. We listened and we looked hard! We made diagnoses. We sat with our patients, or stood by them—literally and in the way the term suggests! We were struggling against the great foe, the awesome antagonist—'Mr. Death,' one of my medical school teachers called him!"

I thought of Dr. Williams, saying those words, late in his life, as he himself was waging such a struggle, and I thought of "Mr. Death" as I looked at the photographs the reader will soon react to with curiosity, surprise, even shock. They make plain the grimness of the contest waged by so many for so long on behalf of time, as much time as possible among the living. In picture after picture the same theme asserts itself for our contemplation: life in all its vulnerability and jeopardy, in all its pain and suffering, trying hard to keep alive its flame, despite the constant winds of darkness that threaten to extinguish it. Amid such solemn contention, I see doctors, nurses, and others who work with them trying to show their patients (and themselves) what is known, what might work to make them better, to bring back (relative) health to those in pain. "It was tough back then," Dr. Williams told me; but it was clear he was not eager for pity when he added forcefully: "But it was also a great privilege we all had—to figure out what was bothering our patients, and to try to be of comfort to them, to hear them out, and sometimes add our two cents, as we talked about what was happening, and what might happen. Lots of stories exchanged! Lots of emotion expressed (and not only by the patients) while we went through our [medical] routines."

Those routines have their documentation in these pages: the continuities and discontinuities of a profession's historical life. Although much has changed since the dawn of the twentieth century, a great deal has remained constant. We still measure blood pressure, peer into microscopes, attend our patients with our ears, and with the "ears" of our stethoscopes. We still knock at knees with our neurological hammers and, yes, have our own grim, admonitory signs posted in hospitals, on billboards, or on the walls of our offices. AIDS has replaced tuberculosis and syphilis as a source of widespread, publicly announced concern—though both of those diseases, for all our antibiotic prowess, have yet to be vanquished. Our swift ambulances have made the horse-drawn kind seem quaint, and our mastery of antisepsis prompts our incredulity as we look at what once took place in the name of surgery, in the name of "hygienic medicine." Still, as these pictures tell us, and as Dr. Williams knew to remind us, there was great dignity in that medical past: the courage of the living—linking arms, joining hands (doctors and patients together) in their hope against hope for a respite from "Mr. Death." The chronicle ahead reminds us not only of what once was, but of what still is, and will always be—our nature as we keep struggling with increasing ingenuity to hold back, as far as possible, that time when the last breath is taken.

—Robert Coles

CHAPTER ONE

THE SEARCH FOR A CURE

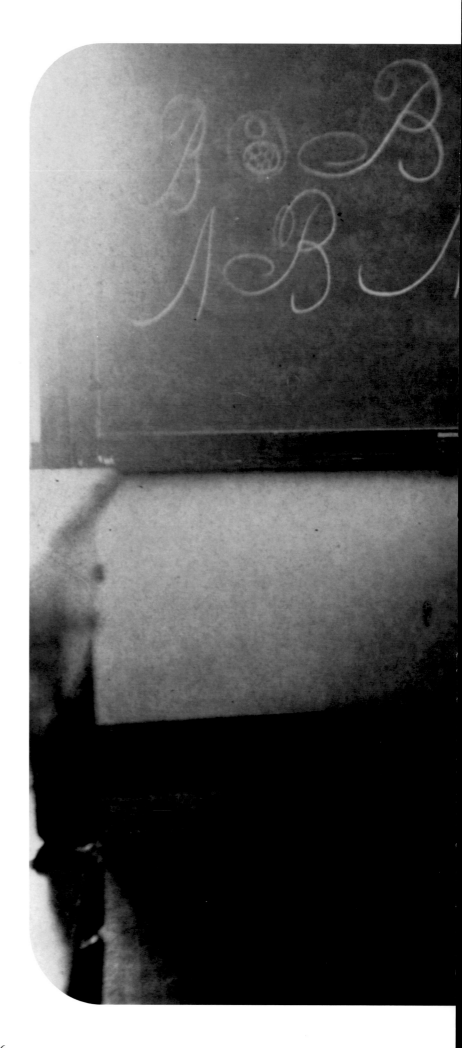

THE TWENTIETH CENTURY WAS LESS THAN TWO DECADES AWAY, AND THE PRESIDENT OF THE UNITED STATES WAS JAMES A. GARFIELD, A DEFT REPUBLICAN POLITICIAN WHO MIGHT HAVE MADE A GOOD CHIEF EXECUTIVE. BUT ON JULY 2, 1881, LESS THAN SIX MONTHS INTO HIS FIRST TERM, HE WAS SHOT BY A NE'ER-DO-WELL NAMED CHARLES JULIUS GUITEAU, WHO SAID GOD HAD CHOSEN HIM TO DO THE DEED.

Garfield, as it turned out, had the great misfortune of being shot a few years too soon. What happened over the next eight days, in fact, could serve as a paradigm of what was wrong with medicine in those days and what had to go right before it could transform itself from a dubious art to a reputable and indeed marvelous science. As Garfield lay on the floor, the doctors' immediate concern was to find the bullet. Even before moving him, they began digging around in the wound with fingers still soiled by a day's work and with instruments that had not been washed, much less sterilized. Garfield, who was conscious, knew he was in serious trouble. "I thank you, doctor," he said when one of his physicians offered him hope, "but I am a dead man."

During the eighty days it took the President to die, the nation followed his case with anxiety. Garfield was operated on twice, once without anesthetic, as doctors continued their effort to find the vexatious bullet. Again and again, his wounds were probed with unwashed hands. His health rose and fell. Alexander Graham Bell was called in to try to find the elusive bullet with a device resembling a twentieth-century mine detector. He, too, failed. Every known cure was attempted. The poor President even received nutrient enemas, of something like eggnog, to build strength.

———————

Circa 1890—*Major advances in basic science in the nineteenth century paved the way for a revolution in medicine. "Pure" research, born in university centers like the pathology laboratories (right) of Johns Hopkins University created a dynamic climate for experimentation and reform that led to a "golden age" of discoveries.*

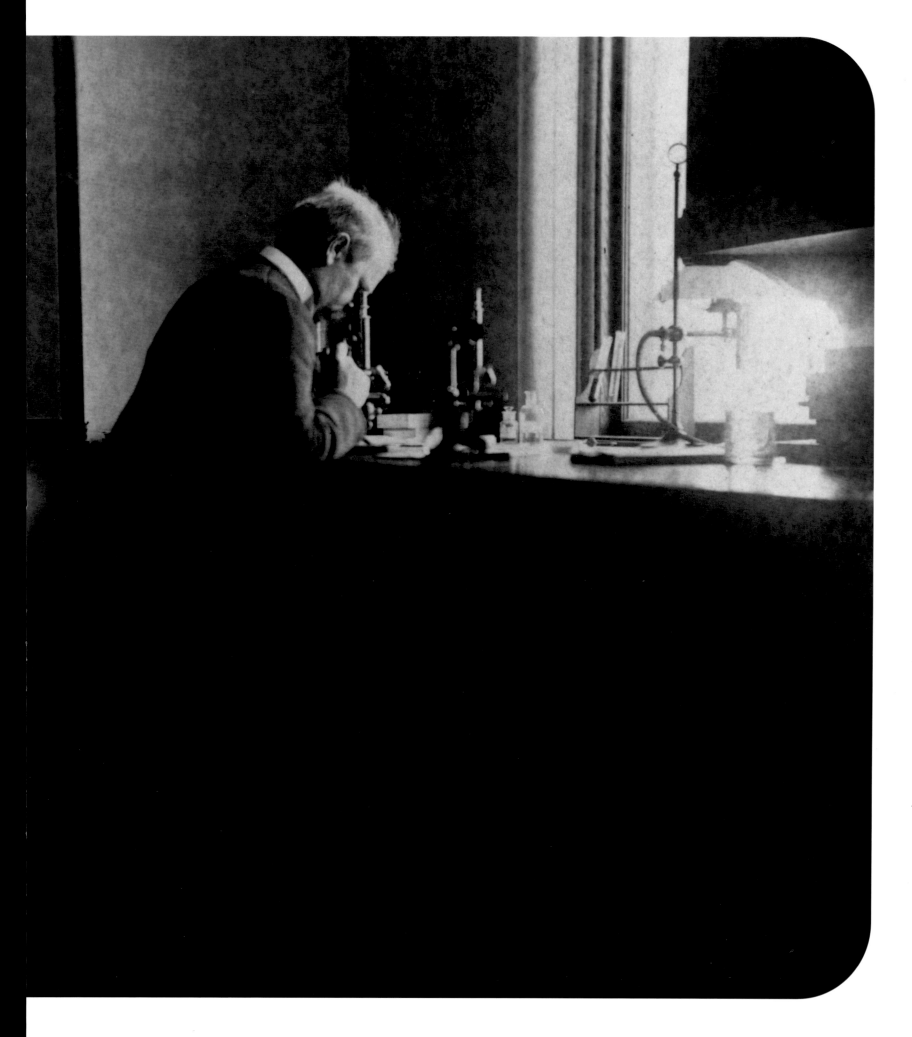

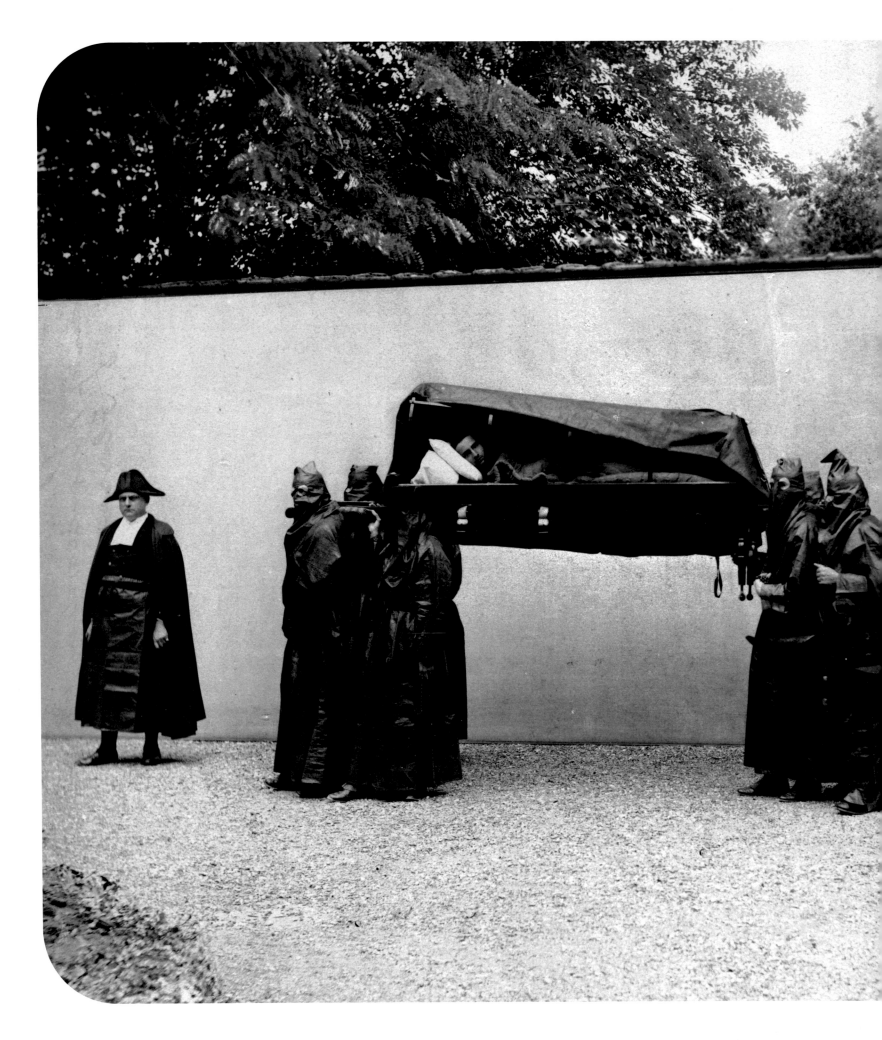

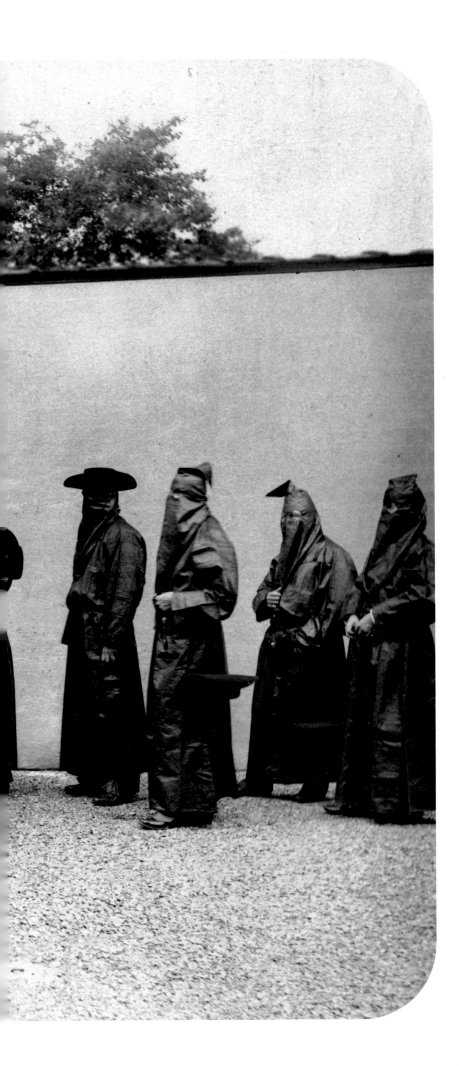

Late in the summer, despite his chief physician's prognosis that the President was going to recover, Garfield died. The immediate cause of death remains a matter of debate, but the dirty fingers, the dirty instruments, and the infection that followed have always been the main targets of the blame. Even the assassin, caught on the spot and later hanged, denied that he had actually killed Garfield. "The doctors did that," Guiteau said. "I simply shot at him."

What Garfield desperately required was a strong dose of medicine. But the period just before and after the turn of the twentieth century was characterized not so much by an abrupt shift toward medical enlightenment as by a gentle arc away from ignorance and superstition. The X ray was developed in 1895. Pierre and Marie Curie discovered radium in 1898. Aspirin appeared in 1899. The Yellow Fever Commission began its seminal work in 1900. And the American hospital began to assume the role it retained for the next one hundred years as a center for learning as well as healing.

This great progress took place against a backdrop of misplaced confidence and outright quackery. Throughout the nineteenth century, a near obsessive reverence for clean air and pure food had taken hold, along with a vague but intense belief in sanitation that would effectively thwart the spread of plagues. Still, in Europe as well as in the United States, bloodletting and purging were common practices. And as late as 1887, a southern doctor, one D. R. Fox, reported that he had treated a woman at childbirth by bleeding her of eighty ounces of blood, dosing her with castor oil, purging her with an enema, and causing her to vomit every two hours—all that within a period of twenty-four hours. Through these ministrations, he reported to his local medical society, she was "restored to health in about four weeks."

But now, at the turn of the century, the field of medicine was about to enter a golden period so productive that more would be learned about the enemies of health and how to combat them in just three generations than had been learned in all the previous millennia humankind had inhabited this planet.

In the late 1880s, the life expectancy of a female was forty-four years. Today, it is nearly eighty. In one spectacular battle after another—against cholera, tuberculosis, yellow fever, syphilis— early twentieth-century medicine achieved its major victories. In 1889, the leading causes of death were consumption, pneumonia, infant cholera, measles, cancer, typhoid fever, diphtheria, croup, bronchitis, whooping cough, and scarlet fever. Only one (cancer) can still spark the same fear it once did.

———

Circa 1900—*The somberly dressed members of the Brotherhood of the Bleeding Heart transport a plague victim in Florence, Italy. The arrival of the bubonic plague—the dread Black Death, borne by rats and fleas—was a terrifying event that affected virtually everyone in the community where it struck.*

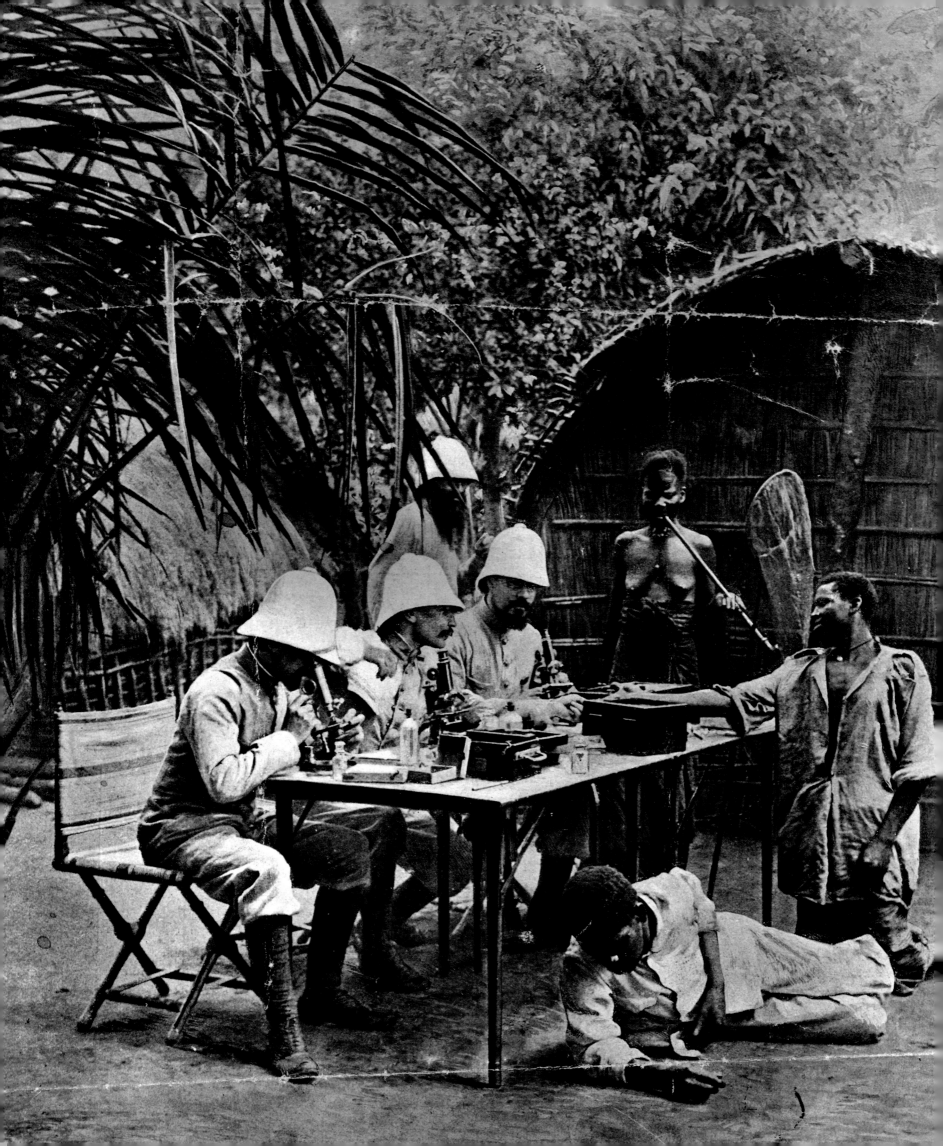

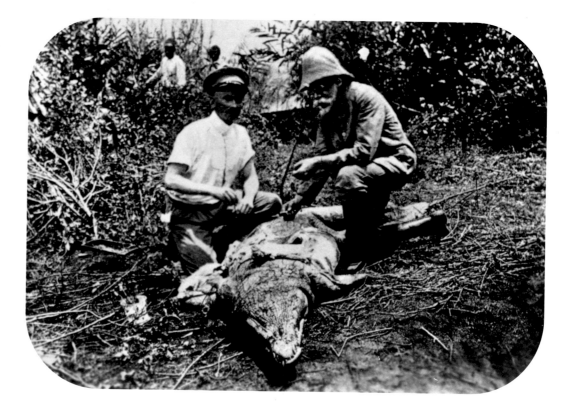

1897—In Africa on the trail of a sleeping sickness cure, Robert Koch (opposite and top right) (1843-1910) meets the tsetse fly. Koch spent much of his life searching for the cause and cure of disease. With Louis Pasteur, he was one of the great pioneers in bacteriology. Koch was the first to link specific bacteria to specific illnesses and to develop methods to culture and identify the organisms. Today, medical science still turns to the famous Koch postulates by which he tested the validity of any theory about how a disease is transmitted: the suspected organism should be found in each case of the disease; it should not be found in other diseases; it should be isolated; it should be cultured; an inoculation employing the organism should produce the same disease; and it should be recoverable in the inoculated animal.

1906—The great hunter of disease, Robert Koch, is seen on an expedition in Africa with F. K. Kleine, dissecting a crocodile (top right). Koch's discovery in 1882 of the tuberculosis bacillus—and of the cholera bacillus on an 1883 trip to Egypt and India—paved the way for the successful assault on two of mankind's most pernicious enemies.

Circa 1906-1907—(bottom right) Dr. Alexandre-Emile Yersin (1863-1943) was a physician whose wanderlust brought him into the mainstream of medical history. The Swiss-born doctor and teacher was serving aboard sailing ships on cruises to the Orient when he was asked by the colonial government in Indochina to help in an outbreak of the plague ravaging China. In 1894, in Hong Kong, he made the breakthrough: he discovered the cause of this monstrous scourge; the bacterium, Yersinia pestis, *now bears his name. Riding the crest of that fame, he was eventually named director of the Pasteur Institutes in Indochina, where he lived, in Annam, until his death.*

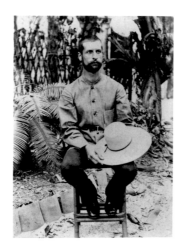

To get the upper hand, medical science had to understand the causes of individual diseases and the courses each one naturally took. The job required the development of whole fields of medicine and research. Bacteriology began to catch on and grow; virology followed. Together, they gave rise to immunology and the modern pharmaceutical industry. And through it all, the new field of epidemiology began to chart the incidence of disease throughout the world and search for critical associations: fat and heart disease, smoking and cancer.

Perhaps most important, medicine would have to become scientific, verifiable, believable. For that to happen would take extraordinary experimentation, and sometimes heroism as well.

THE YELLOW FEVER RIDDLE

Although many of those struck by yellow fever survived, it was nevertheless a killer on a dreadful scale throughout the nineteenth century. The tropical island of Cuba was known to be rife with the disease—deeply unsettling news to American officials as the Spanish-American war progressed in 1898, and they feared greater losses from disease than from battle. By 1900, yellow fever had struck down many Americans in Cuba, even killing officers who lived in far more sanitary conditions than other servicemen. The United States Surgeon General

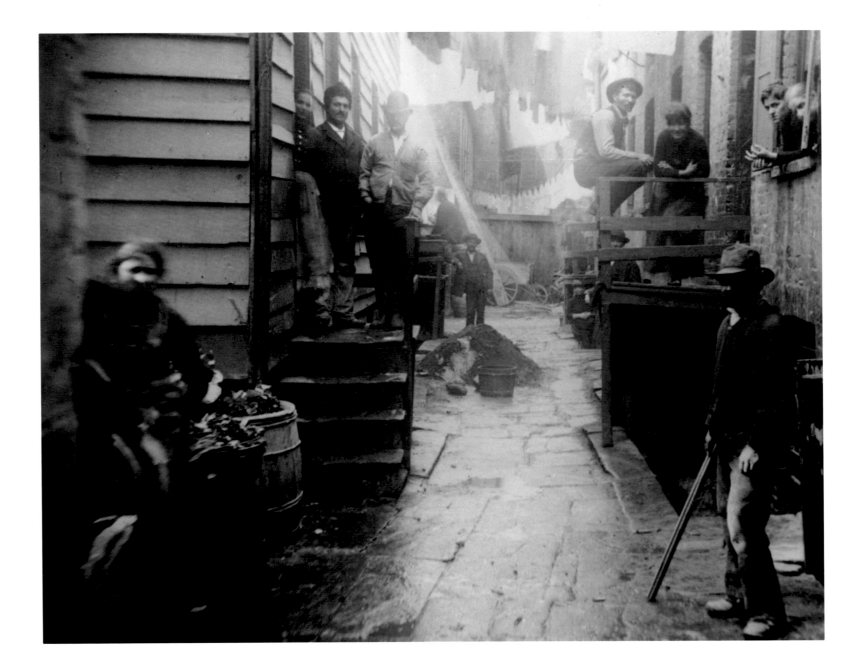

decided to form a commission to go to Cuba and investigate the causes of the disease.

In the medical community, two rival points of view competed for attention. One was that the fever was caused by bacteria, a theory put forward by an Italian bacteriologist, Dr. Giuseppe Sanarelli, who had worked at the Pasteur Institute in Paris. While doing research in Brazil and Uruguay in 1897, he even named the alleged villain: *bacillus icteroides.*

The other theory held that mosquitoes were doing the damage by injecting some unknown toxin that caused the disease. The early evidence that pointed to mosquitoes came mostly from the work of a Cuban physician named Carlos Finlay. It was already known that some parasitic diseases could be spread to human beings by ticks and tsetse flies, and for years the possible culpability of mosquitoes in yellow fever had been a matter of speculation. Finlay

Circa 1910— *The notorious "Bandit's Alley" was one of New York's worst slum areas. The squalor in which its tenement dwellers lived eventually led to a wave of health reforms. Politicians joined with sanitation activists to attack poverty and blight and create a powerful and effective public health movement.*
Photographed by R. H. Lawrence

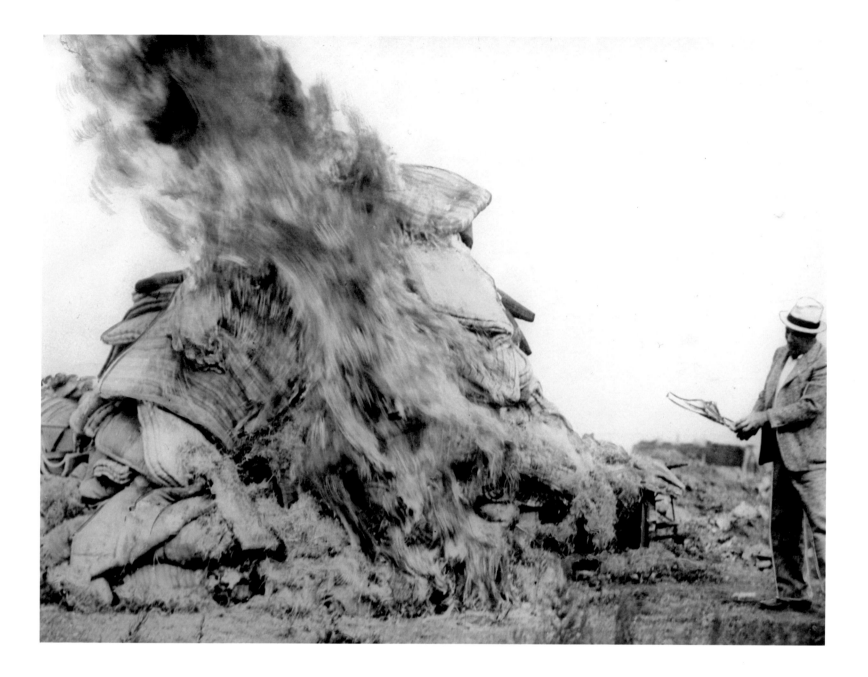

Circa 1918—*The fire this time… In the absence of other proven methods to thwart a devastating contagion, supposedly contaminated mattresses are burned during an influenza clean-up. In 1918 and 1919, Spanish flu, one of the many virulent strains of the epidemic, attacked five million Americans and left half a million dead.*

set about trying to prove it. He got close, but he was unable to achieve one crucial experimental step: to demonstrate the actual transmission of the disease to human subjects through mosquito bites. Some of his volunteers, once bitten, developed fevers but not the disease itself. Later it was discovered that Finlay used the mosquitoes in experiments before the insects were fully infectious.

Despite this initial failure, the Surgeon General's commission—comprising Major Walter Reed, Dr. Aristides Agramonte, Dr. James Carroll, and Dr. Jesse Lazear—would eventually discard the bacteria hypothesis and champion the mosquito answer. They went to Finlay, obtained mosquito larvae from him, and then placed the hatched mosquitoes on the bodies of infected people so that the insects could gorge on the infectious agent. Next they came to a courageous decision: they decided to let themselves be bitten by the infected mosquitoes. Carroll infected himself with the virus first. Lazear, seeing Carroll's success in becoming ill, needed to verify that the mosquito bites were the cause of the symptoms. He took the very mosquito that had felled his colleague and applied it, along with three others, to the arm of a volunteer named Dean, who also became sick—though he eventually recovered. Lazear wrote to his wife: "I rather think I am on the track of the real germ but nothing must be said as yet, not even a hint. I have not mentioned it to a soul." It was his last letter to her—after letting himself be bitten, he died of yellow fever on September 25, twelve days after beginning his experiment.

Eventually, the whole world knew. The discovery that yellow fever was caused not by bacteria but by a disease carried by mosquitoes led to campaigns of massive fumigation in mosquito-infested areas. This in turn made possible the completion of the Panama Canal and resulted in the eradication of the disease in the United States by 1907. Every tropical area in the world benefited from this discovery, and the air of meticulous experimentation that surrounded the conquest of yellow fever not only represented the new scientific mentality in medicine but also contributed to it.

Was Diet the Culprit?

Pellagra is a virtually forgotten disorder today. (We might wonder whether leukemia or multiple sclerosis will be words without meaning a hundred years from now.) But in the 1700s the "disease of the three D's," as it was called (dementia, dermatitis, and diarrhea), affected a substantial number of Europeans. In the United

1914—*The missionaries of cleanliness fanned out through the world in the early part of the century. In this Lewis Hine photograph, a Red Cross nurse in Skoplie, Turkey, teaches mothers how to tend to their children. Hine's pictures—published in newspapers, social welfare journals, on posters and flyers—were weapons in the arsenal of public education.*

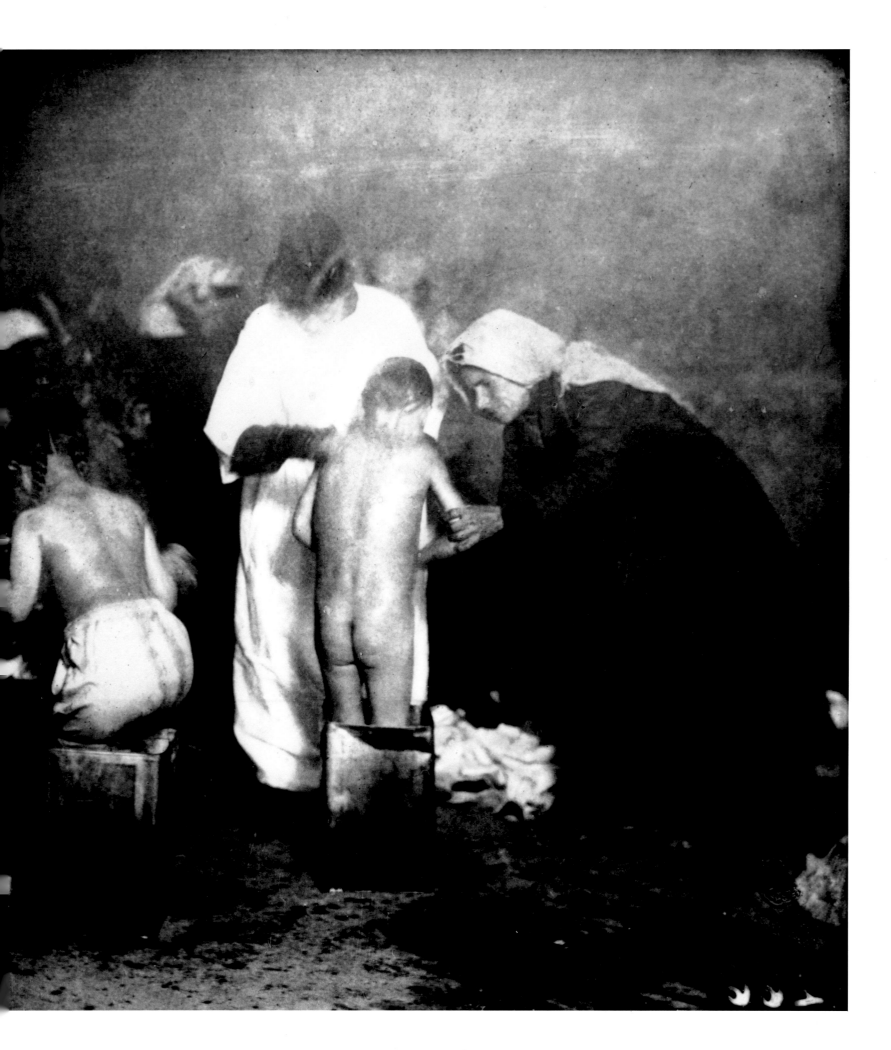

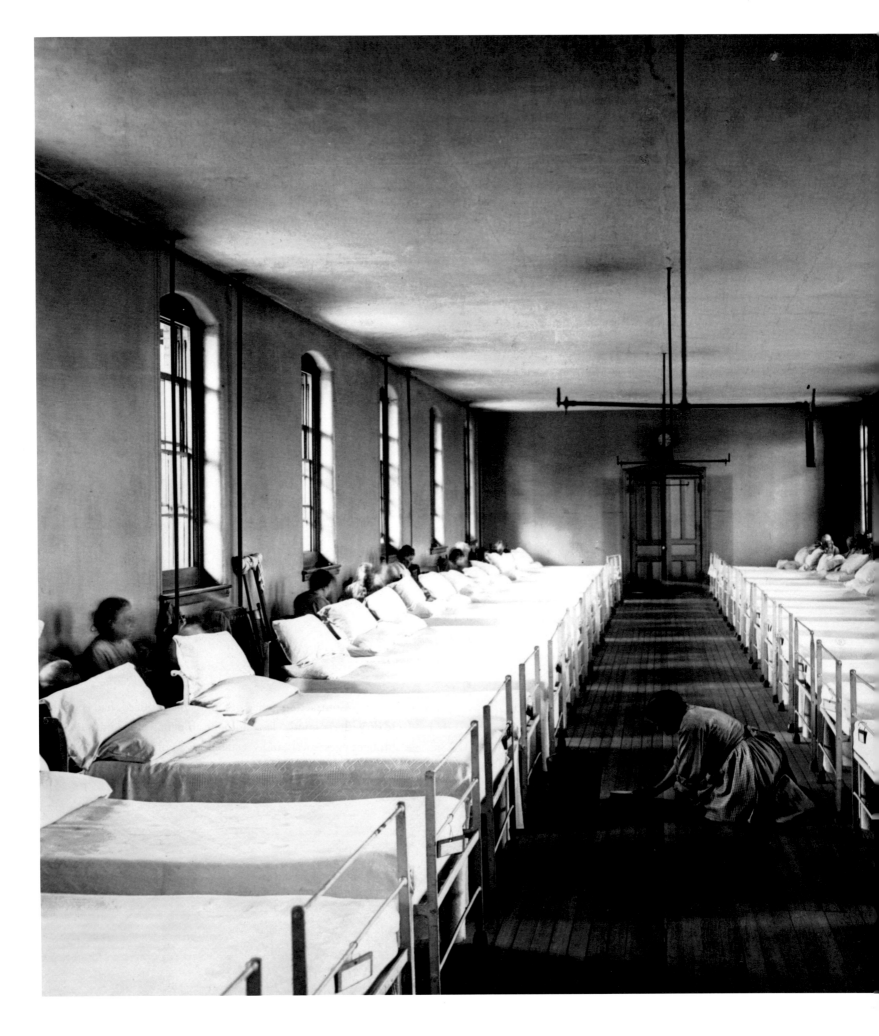

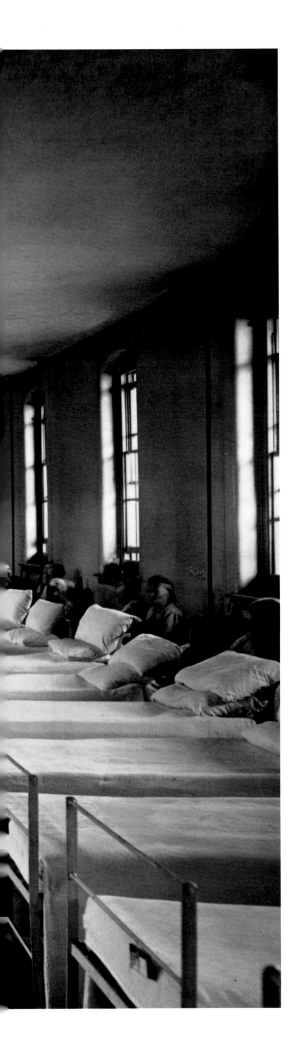

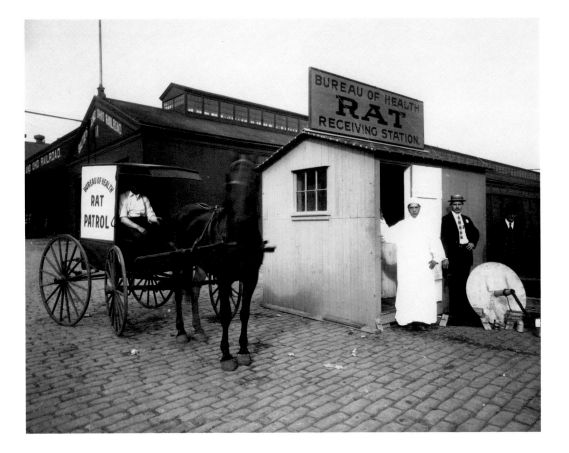

States in the nineteenth century, it brought misery to places such as asylums, where people were confined, and to many poor communities in the South.

At the turn of the century, a time when bacteria were blamed for many diseases, pellagra was generally presumed to be an infectious disease. Some people, however, suspected it might be hereditary, while still others thought it might be dietetic in some mysterious way. Among the latter was Dr. Joseph Goldberger of the U.S. Public Health Service. In 1914, Dr. Goldberger was named to head a federal project to investigate the disease.

Contracting pellagra, Goldberger noticed, had something to do with economic class, since the affluent seemed immune. So he brought eggs, meat, and vegetables to an orphanage in Mississippi and eradicated the disease from one ward while he watched it flourish in another that had not been given the same balanced diet. He reversed the experimental process by producing pellagra in a group

---

Circa 1900—*(left) Outpatient ward in the female barracks, City Home, New York. The almshouse, also known as the poorhouse, was a predecessor of the hospital, but its patients were the poor, the orphaned, and the enfeebled.*

Circa 1914—*(above) Rat patrol, Philadelphia. A small extermination industry grew up around the effort to fight typhus by eliminating its carrier, the rat. The most popular methods included building and setting rat traps and dusting rat runs with poison.*

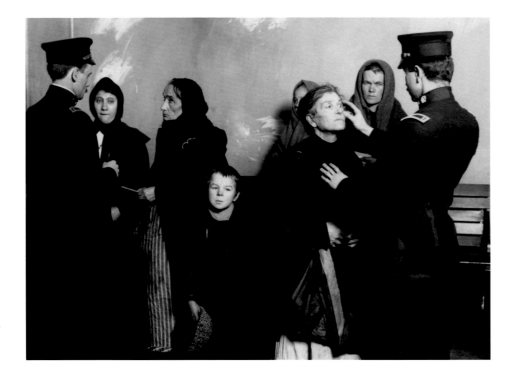

of prisoners (experimental subjects were not as sensitively treated then as they are today) by putting them on a diet low in protein but otherwise healthy.

Goldberger next had to prove that the disease could not be transmitted from one human being to another. To do that he concocted a hideous series of experiments. Like Carroll in the case of yellow fever, Goldberger courageously placed himself among those medical scientists who used their own bodies as testing grounds. Dr. Lawrence K. Altman, the medical correspondent for The New York Times, describes the research in his fine 1987 book about self-experimentation, *Who Goes First?:*

"About a fifth of an ounce of blood drawn from a patient with a moderately acute first attack of pellagra was injected into the forty-two-year-old doctor's left shoulder and into the shoulder of another volunteer, Dr. George A. Wheeler. Wheeler then rubbed secretions taken from the nose and mouth of the pellagra patient into Goldberger's nose and mouth. Goldberger returned the favor. Nothing untoward happened."

Goldberger could now certify that pellagra was not communicable, but rather caused by a deficient diet. Though cancer ended Goldberger's career in 1929 before he could find the specific cause of the disease he had been pursuing for so long, Dr. Conrad A. Elvehjem of the University of Wisconsin discovered in 1929 that a specific nutrient, nicotinic acid—or niacin—could cure pellagra.

The experiments with pellagra marked one of the major advances in understanding the role of diet in sickness and health. In 1912, the British biochemist Sir Frederick Gowland Hopkins described certain essential substances in food as "accessory factors" to the diet. A Polish-born biochemist working in England, Casimir

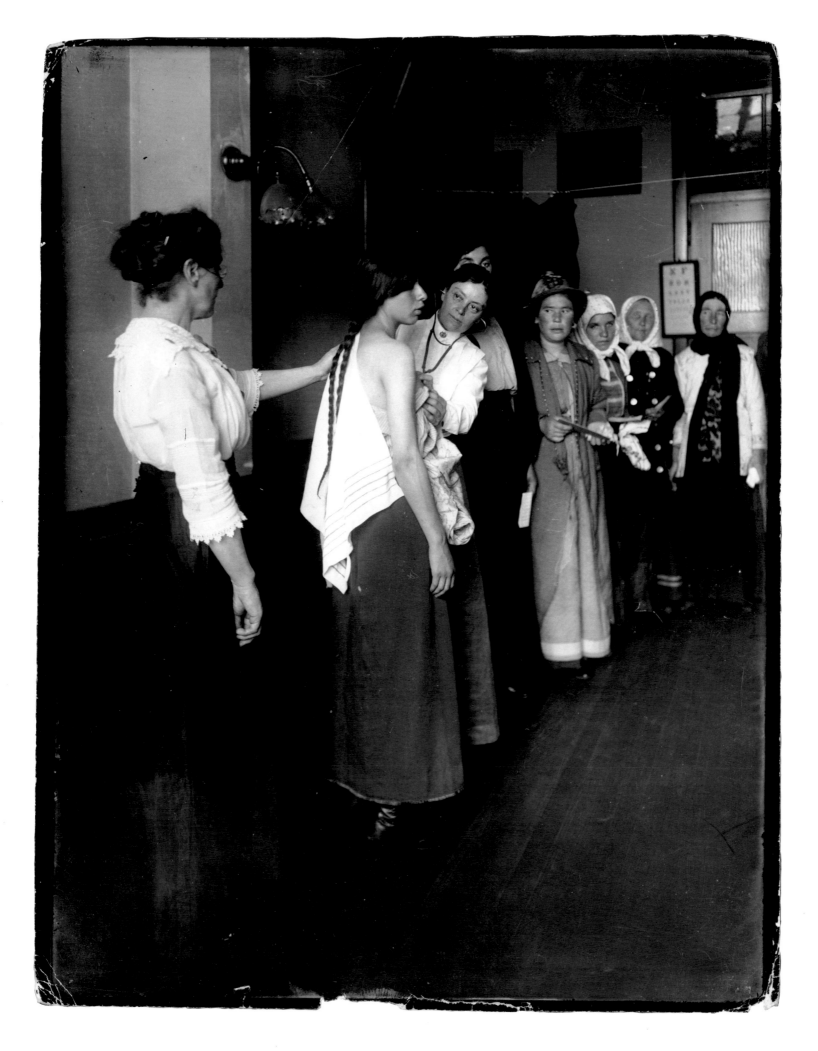

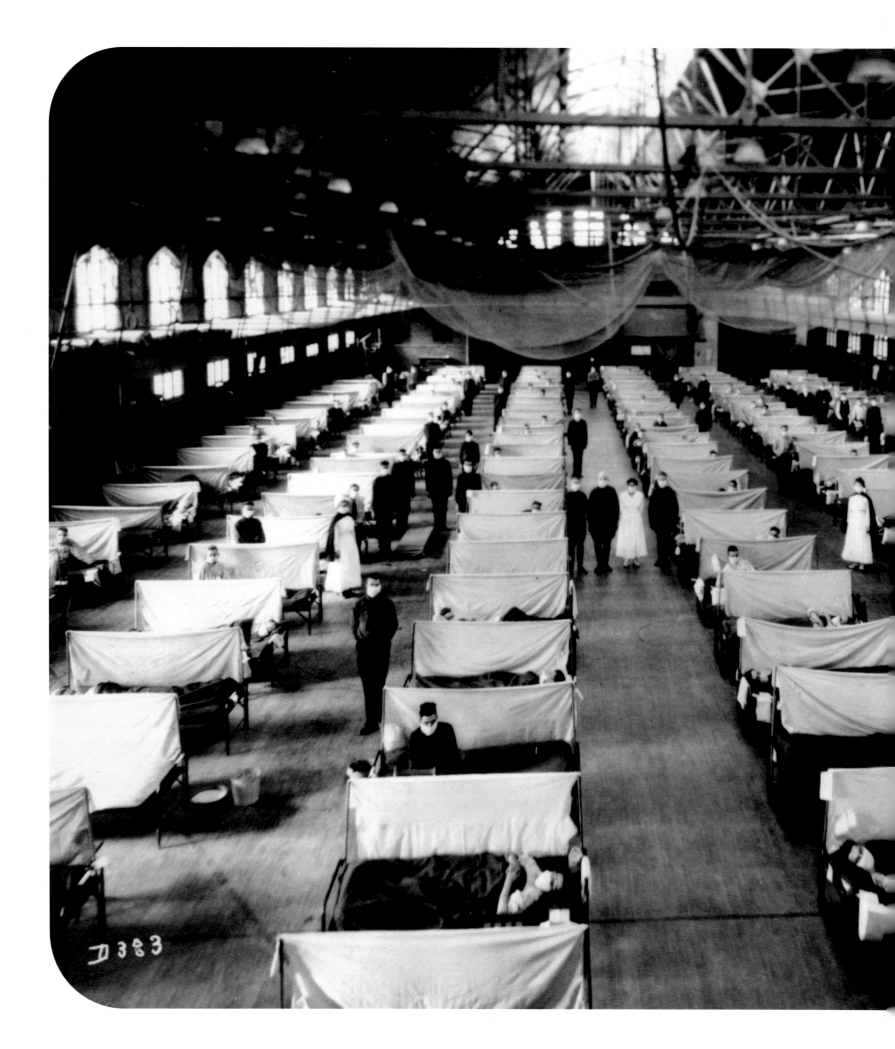

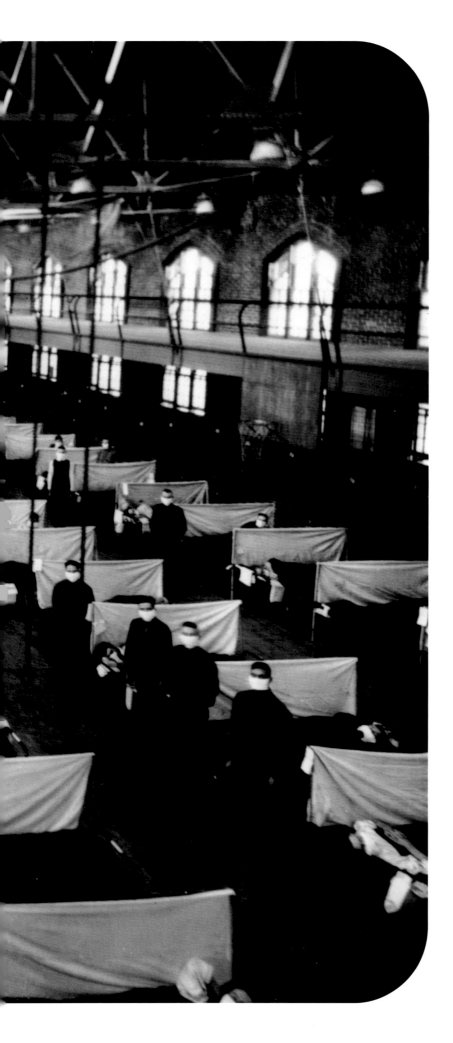

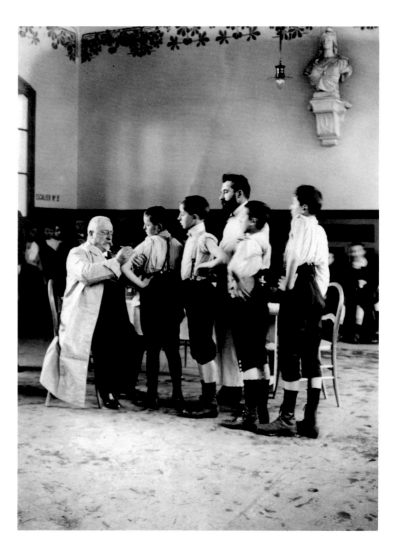

Funk, came to the conclusion that all of them contained a nitrogen component called an amine. He named the substances "vital amines," or "vitamines." It later turned out that some of them did not contain nitrogen, so the term was altered slightly to "vitamins," the name they carry to this day.

As the vitamins revealed themselves one by one, food was fortified—flour, bread, and milk in particular—gradually turning the deficiency diseases such as pellagra and beriberi into historical stories of medical triumph. Today these advances in nutrition are taken for granted; common supermarket staples are likely to carry the word "enriched," designating, among other things, that they may contain niacin. Pellagra is all but no more. *(continued on page 27)*

Circa 1918—*(left) The Spanish flu advanced unchecked despite a huge public health effort. Congress was forced to allocate $1 million to the Public Health Service to hire doctors and nurses to care for the sick. Massive infirmaries, such as this one at the Iowa State University gymnasium, did what they could to cope with the avalanche of patients.*

Circa 1900—*(above) In France, where Pasteur's work was an impetus for the modern vaccine, schoolchildren were immunized against smallpox.*

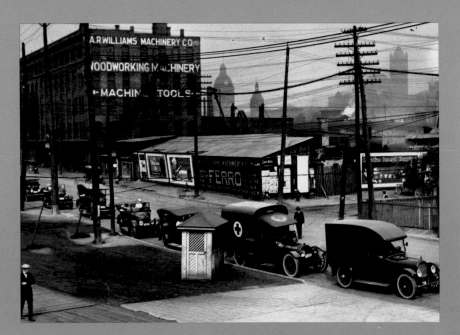

Following the Sun

For youngsters afflicted with the acute and chronic diseases of childhood, doctors could do little more than prescribe rest, healthy food and exposure to fresh air. At the turn of the century hospitals and other institutions were involved in organizing fresh air camps.

Ambulances like those pictured above (circa 1920) ferried children from Toronto's Hospital for Sick Children to a lakeside wharf where the *Luella, (right)* continued on to an island retreat. At the idyllic Lakeside Home for Little Children at Gibraltar Point on Toronto Island, children were coaxed back to health with ministrations of air and sunshine.

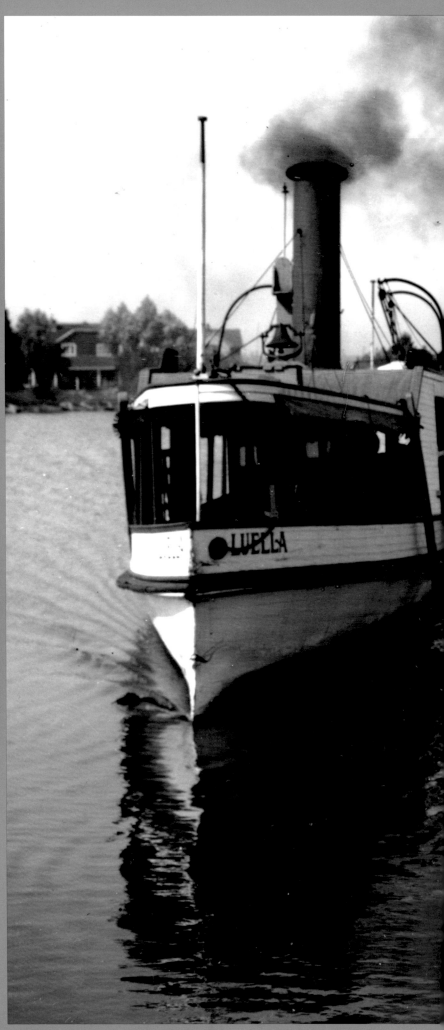

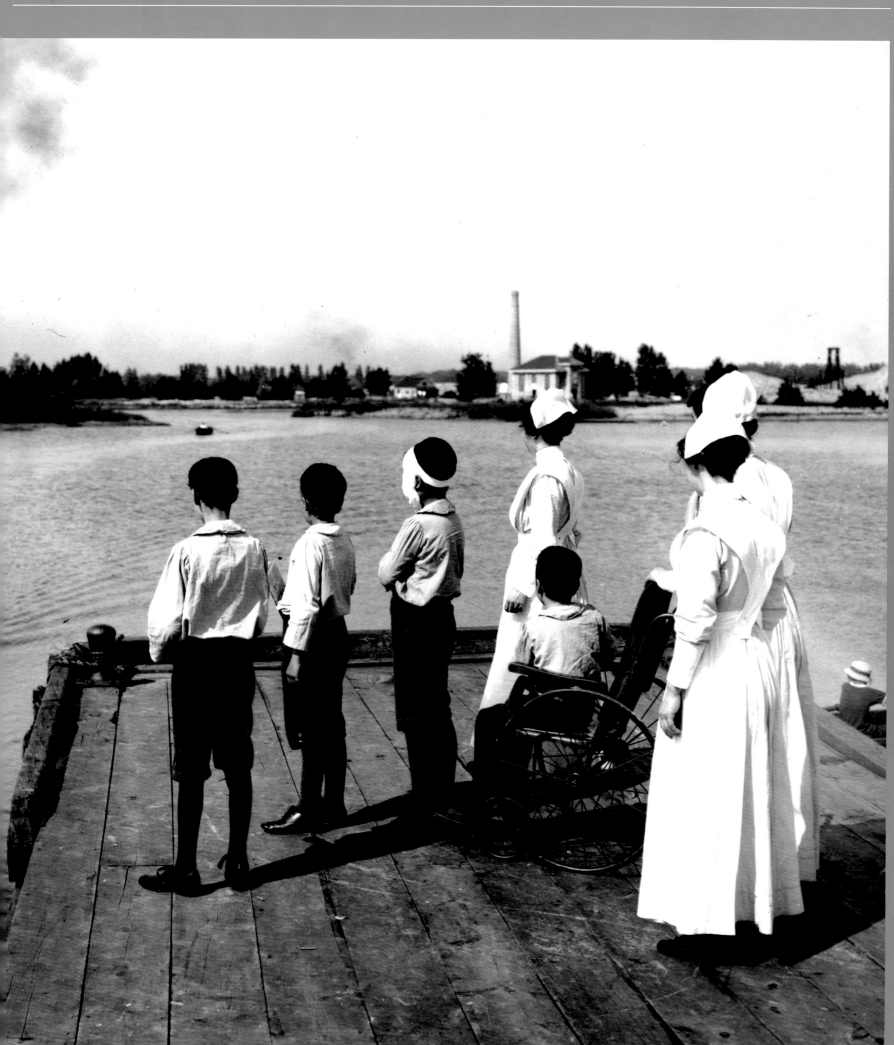

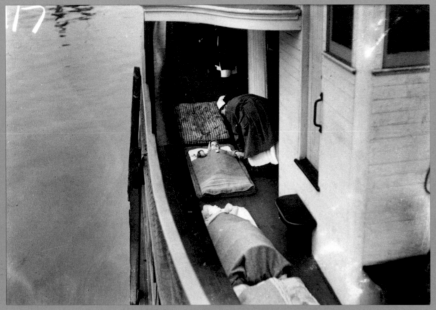

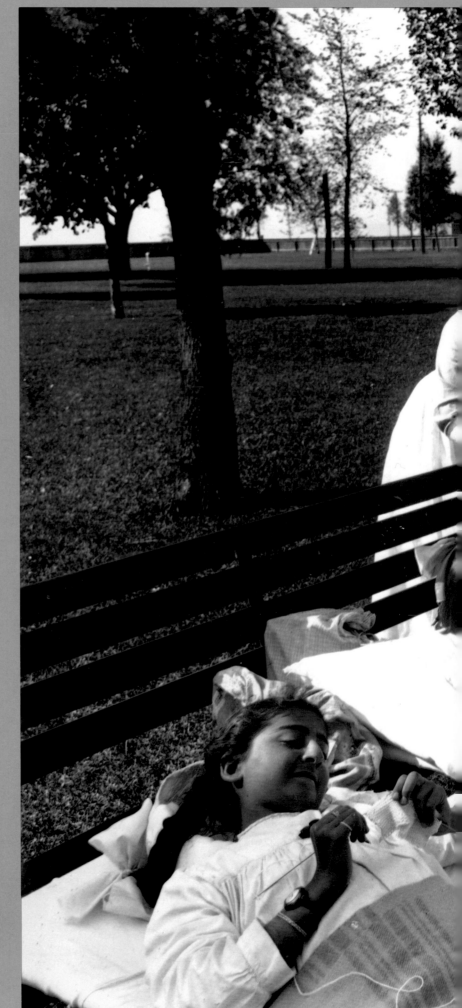

Fresh air camps were considered essential in the treatment of the acute, contagious diseases that plagued children before preventive inoculations were discovered. The camps were considered essential for the treatment of "consumption," as tuberculosis was once called. The children took advantage of the fresh air during the boat ride to camp *(above)*. Camps encouraged children to rest and engage in only very light activities, such as knitting sweaters for soldiers *(right)*.

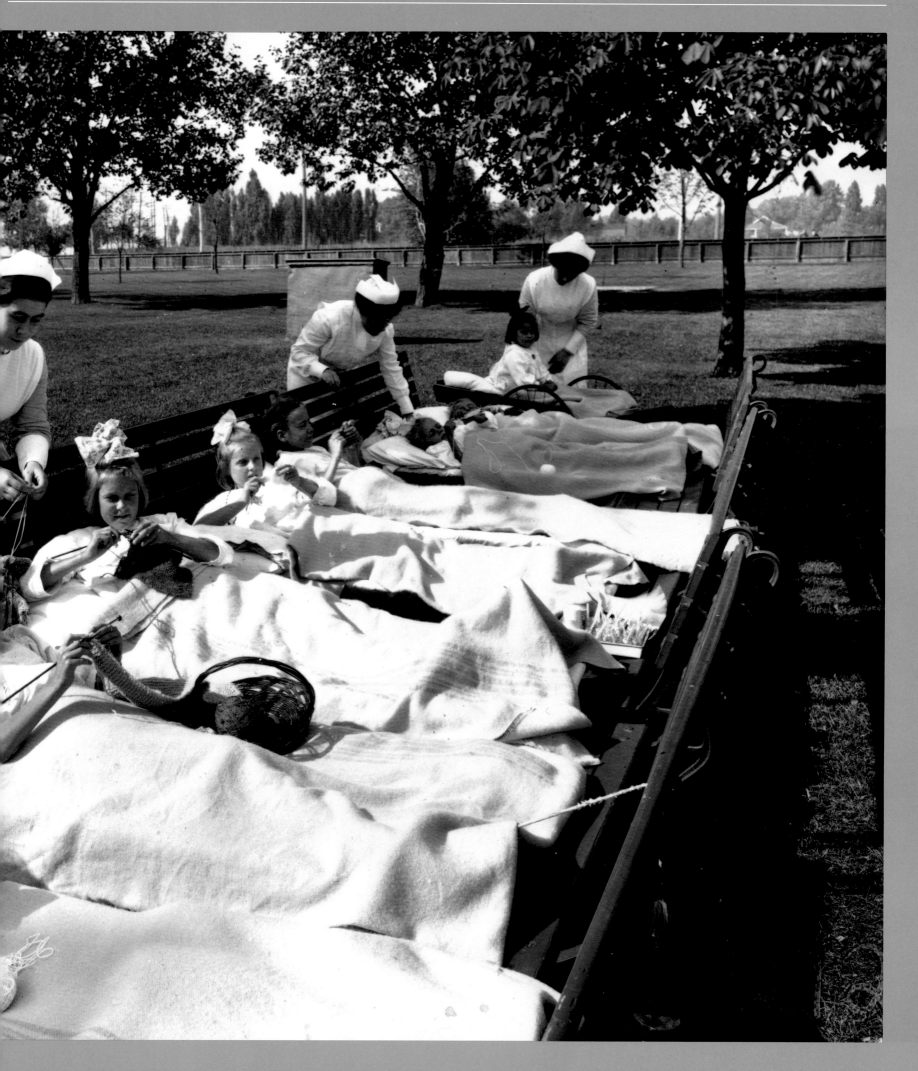

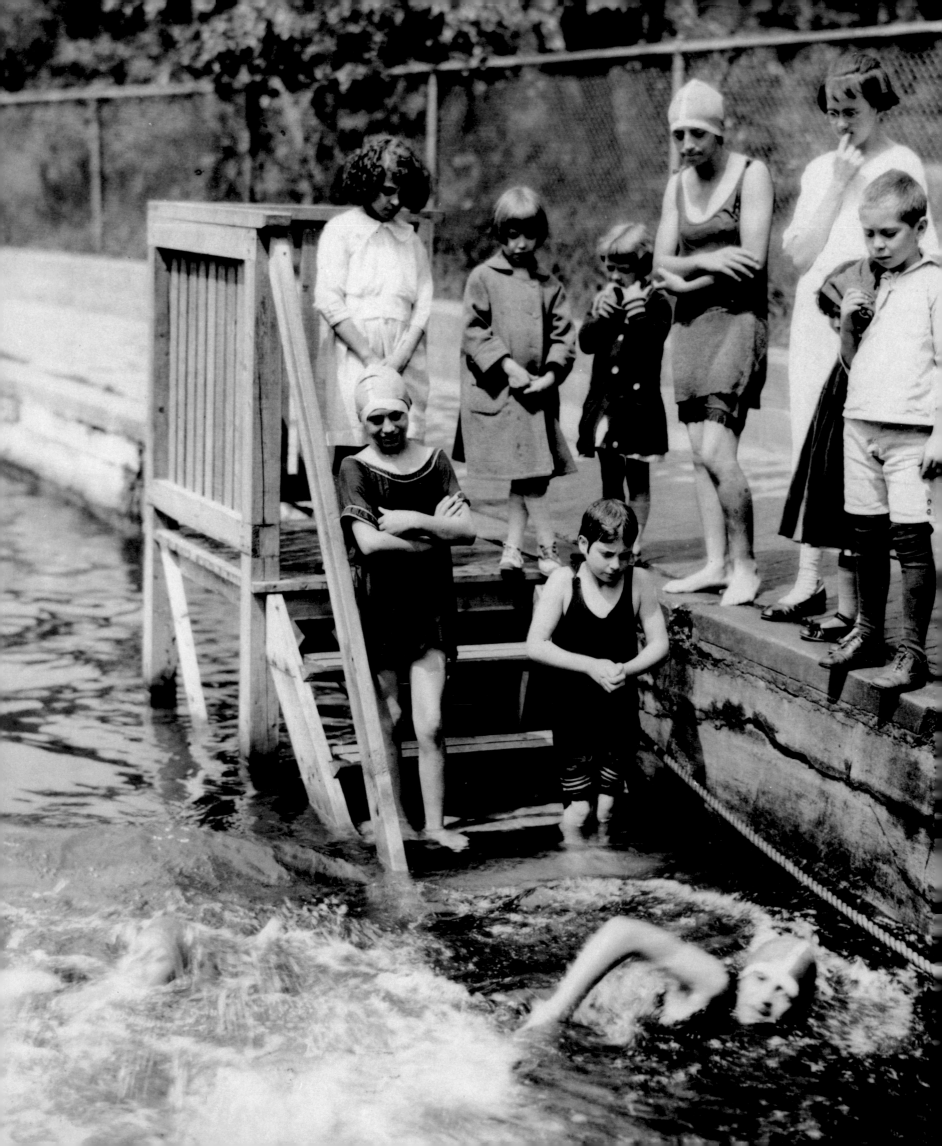

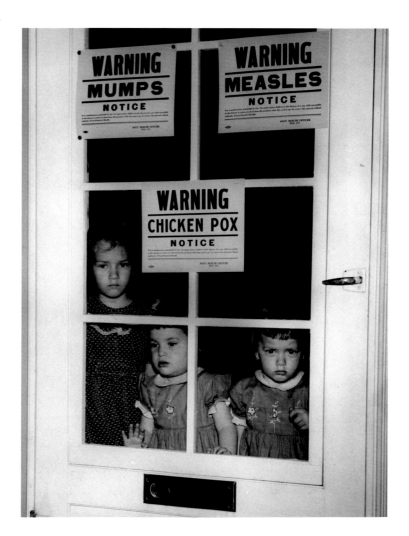

1921—*(opposite) A bit chilly, but probably a character builder: youngsters at the Goodhue Farm, a division of Bellevue Hospital, confront the water. Despite its proximity to Manhattan, the farm on Staten Island was a world away from the grime and crowding of New York. Photographed by A. T. Beals.*

1953—*(above) Even at mid-century, childhood was an extraordinarily dangerous time: mumps, measles, and chicken pox, the triple threat. Photographed by Tom Merryman.*

Still with us, though, is a kind of hangover from celebrating the discovery of these vital nutrients. There are now thirteen known vitamins, but nutritional medicine men keep trying to push others our way, such as P, or certain new B vitamins with high numbers in the subscript. And the discussion of vitamins has too often been dominated by wishful thinking, as vitamins have sometimes been pushed as offering simple answers to complex problems—cancer, stress, aging. But lately some of the claims have not seemed so farfetched. Recent studies have shown that vitamin C may play a role in preventing some cancers. Vitamin E may well lower the risk of cardiovascular disease. And vitamin K appears central in thwarting osteoporosis. The story of vitamins continues to unfold in a positive way as nutrients become increasingly important in the arsenal of modern medicine.

PREVENTIVE MEDICINES

Vaccination is one of medicine's cleverest tricks: making the body believe it is sick and thus causing it to marshal just the right forces to ward off that particular sickness. The development of this practice stands as a twentieth-century accomplishment, but its roots reach far back into the past. Centuries ago, the Chinese and the Turks knew enough to produce a medicine against smallpox by grinding up the scabs of people with mild cases of the disease. In 1796, Dr. Edward Jenner found he could induce resistance to smallpox by using the vaccinia virus (*vacca* is Latin for cow) to infect people with the relatively mild cowpox. But it was Louis Pasteur, working a century later, who did the research that finally gave the field of immunology the creative boost that would propel it to the forefront of modern medicine. In 1895, Pasteur produced a rabies vaccine without actually realizing that he was enhancing the body's own immune system; he knew only that the vaccine worked.

But what was the infectious agent that vaccines fought? Could it have been a bacterium? In Germany, in 1882, Robert Koch had shown that just such a germ caused tuberculosis. Microscopic parasites with similarities both to plants and animals, bacteria were certainly the cause of much human misery. But they were not to play the starring role in the vaccine story.

The first tantalizing awareness of a virus—a microorganism even stranger than the invisible bacteria and like nothing else ever known before—came in 1898 when Martinus Willem Beijerinick discovered a minuscule living thing he described with a name, "virus," derived from the Latin for poisonous slime. It was not until 1935 that Wendell Stanley, a biochemist at the Rockefeller Institute, identified the protein that marks viruses as singular forms of life. To put it precisely, viruses are not quite alive in the sense that most of us would recognize life. A virus is really no more than a protein bag carrying its own set of genetic instructions. A virus

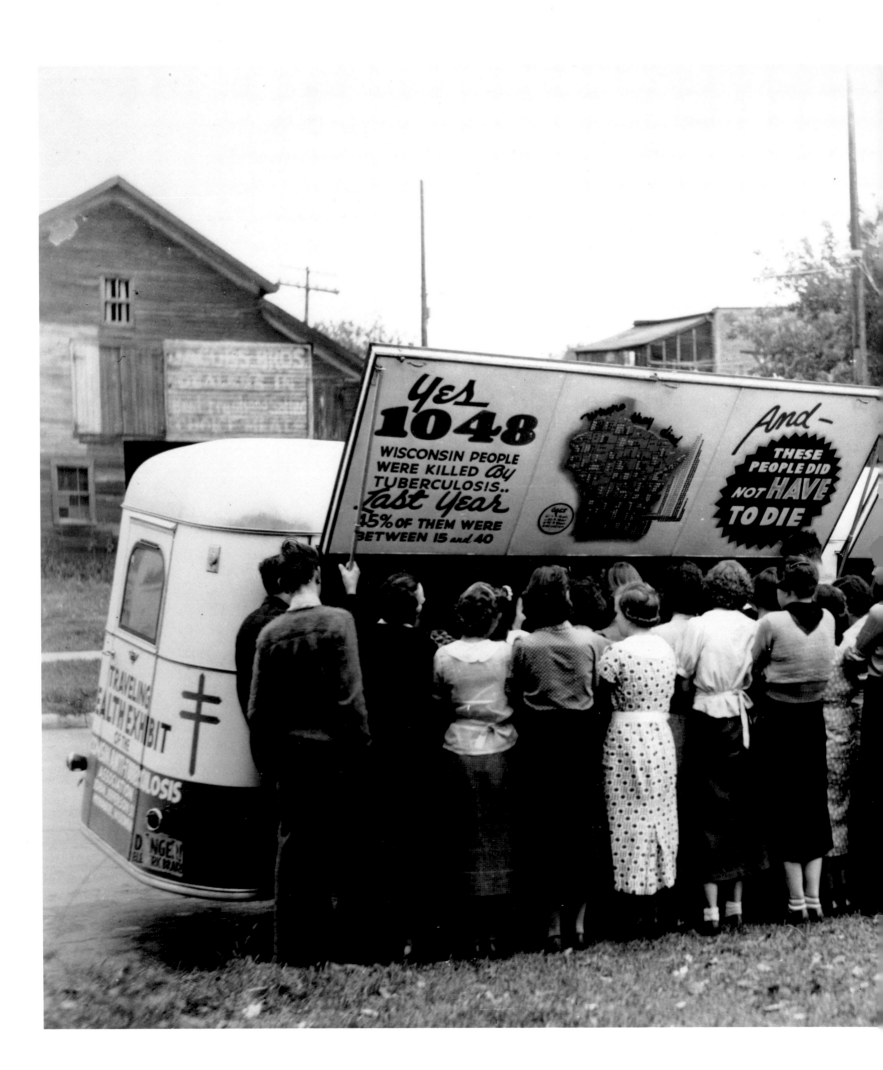

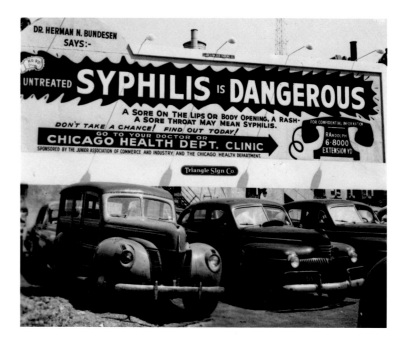

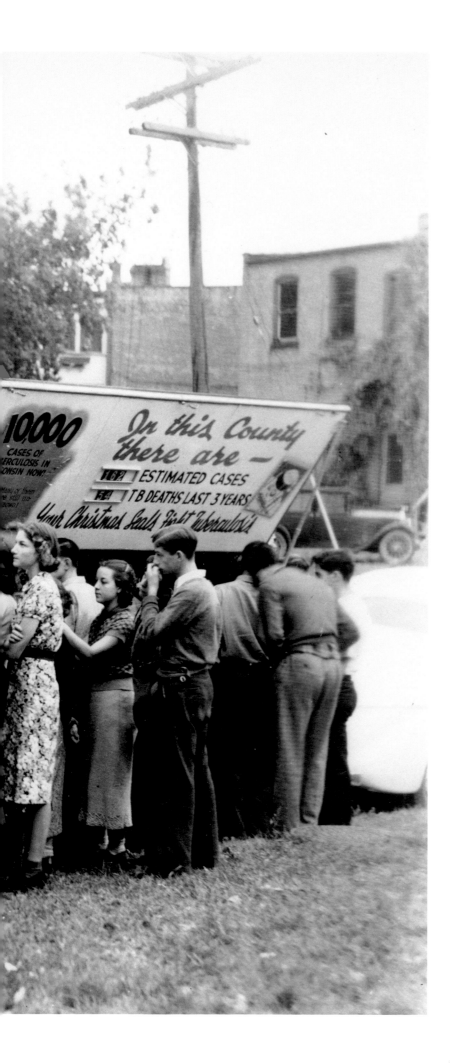

cannot reproduce on its own. It must attach itself to a cell, impregnate the cell with the viral genes, and then, parasite that it is, turn that cell into a reproductive machine for the virus's benefit. The body, for the most part, is able to recognize these viruses as foreign invaders by the signature proteins on their surface. It then attacks them with antibodies and sends killer cells to destroy the cells that have already been infected. If the immune system is overwhelmed by the invasion, the body becomes sick and may die. If the body wins, then its immune system keeps a record of this particular enemy and is better prepared to resist the next time. Sometimes the immunity is lifelong.

Thanks to advances in modern vaccines, measles are nearly gone, and chicken pox, whooping cough, typhoid, and cholera are under control. From a purely psychological point of view, perhaps the biggest vaccine success of the century was the almost total victory over polio, an effort that called upon everything scientists had learned in the new fields of immunology and virology. Polio was thought to be a true childhood plague, a crippler and a destroyer of young lives (though science subsequently proved it did not discriminate on the basis of age). It seemed to come from nowhere in 1916 and was virtually eradicated fifty years later, but only after some first-rate science and a feud long remembered for its bitterness.

Ironically, scientists now believe the catastrophic emer-

Circa 1935—(left) The Wisconsin Anti-Tuberculosis Association's traveling health exhibit was one small player in a huge public education effort that had taken hold throughout much of the world.

Circa 1940—(above) The Wassermann blood test in 1906 meant syphilis could be readily detected. The most effective treatment arrived with the development of penicillin. Until then the disease could be fatal.

gence of polio was caused by the relatively new knowledge about sanitation that had wiped out earlier scourges. Previously, children had become infected with polio at an early age (when the disease tended to be nearly harmless and invisible) and would then achieve lifelong immunity to it. But better sanitary conditions meant polio now struck many more children later in their lives.

The names Salk and Sabin, developers of the vaccines used today, are most commonly attached to the fight against and ultimate conquest of polio. But in the annals of science, a great deal of credit is given as well to the work done forty years earlier by Dr. Alexis Carrel and Dr. John F. Enders. Carrel's work at the Rockefeller Institute demonstrated that living cells could be grown outside the body. He discovered he could take cells from the hearts of chicken embryos and keep them alive indefinitely (some of his early tissue cultures actually survived longer than Carrel, who died in 1944). Carrel received the Nobel Prize for his work in 1912. In the 1940s, this culture technique would pave the way for Enders to make the single most important breakthrough against polio.

Enders, a Harvard virologist, managed to produce the polio virus in test tubes, which meant that the incredibly expensive and relatively unproductive method of producing it in monkey spinal columns could now be bypassed. A copious quantity of virus in some form—either dead or greatly weakened—was needed to gently infect large numbers of people so that their immune systems would produce the antibodies that would protect them in the future. For his development of the test-tube technique that would lead to the manufacture of polio virus, Enders, too, won a Nobel.

Jonas Salk emerged in the mid-forties as a junior scientist with high ambitions. He had worked at the University of Michigan at Ann Arbor for Dr. Thomas Francis, Jr., a virologist studying killed vaccines, and was now attached to the unheralded University of Pittsburgh School of Public Health. Salk agreed to take on a job that other virologists evidently found too tedious. The powerful National Foundation for Infantile Paralysis needed a researcher to run its virus-typing project. Viruses often exist in too many variations to allow the production of an effective vaccine, but polio seemed to be the result of only three viruses. Salk's job was to confirm that this was true by employing a series of repetitive lab studies that would eventually, and laboriously, rule out other possibilities.

With Enders' method for reproducing the virus now available, Salk resolved to go about killing it by the tried-and-true

---

Circa 1952—*At the height of the polio epidemic, American hospitals looked like field units in a war zone except that the wounded were children, not soldiers. In the Los Angeles County Hospital in California the iron lung became synonymous with the grim reality of childhood suffering. Many youngsters required the machine to help them breathe once the virus had damaged cells in their brains and spinal cords.*

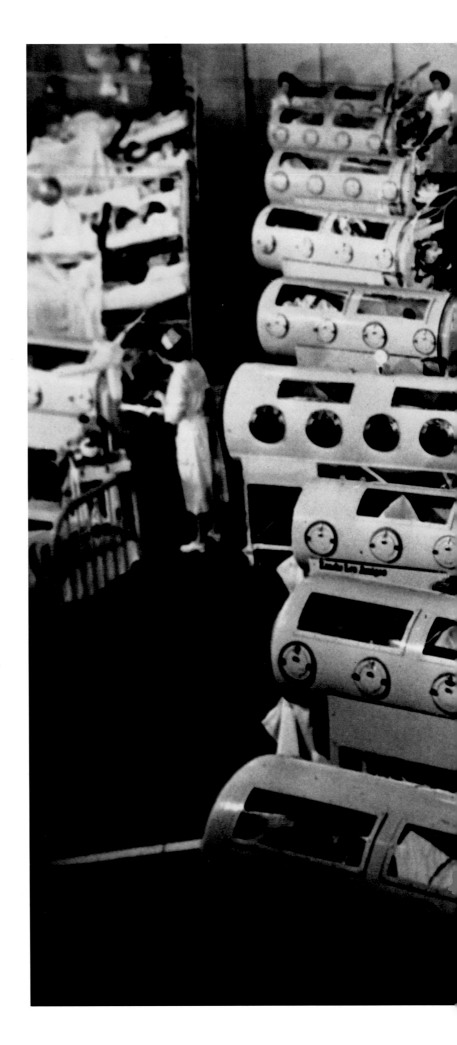

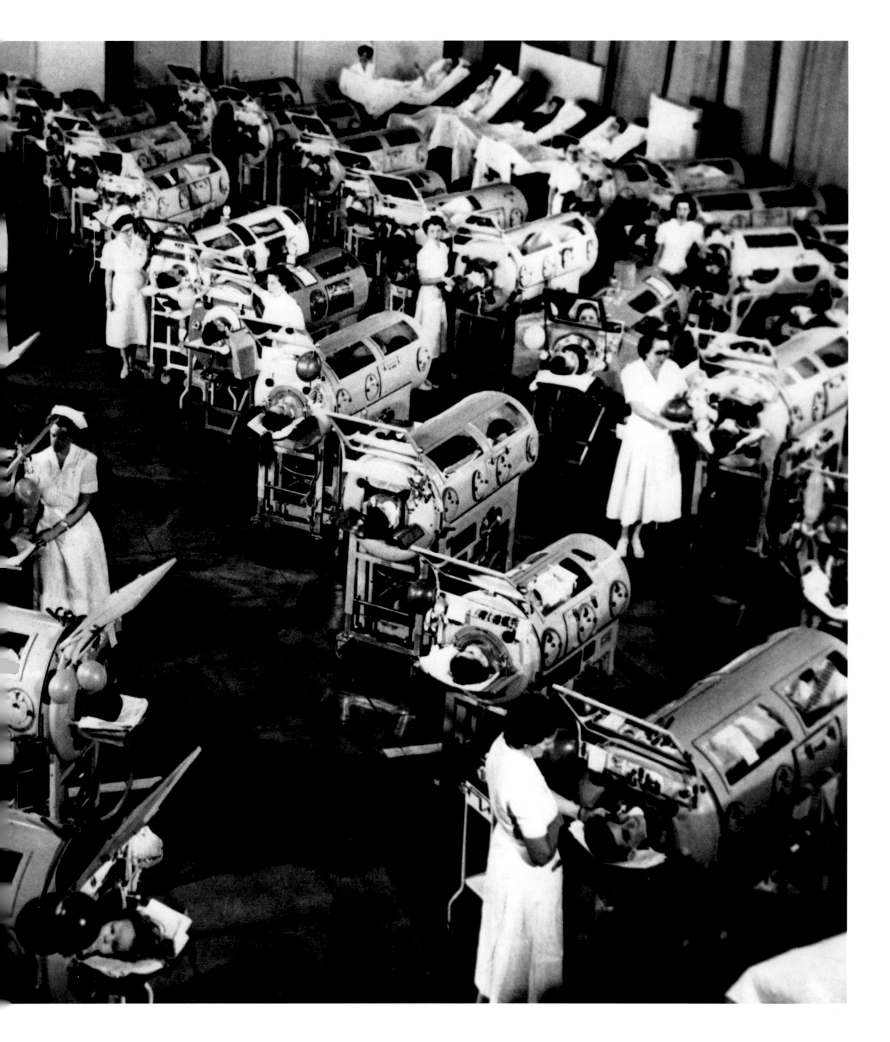

technique of poisoning with formaldehyde. In 1952, a terrible year for polio contagion, Salk was prepared to begin testing. The general belief among scientists was that a killed-virus vaccine could not work as well as a weakened live virus would. They believed that even though the body's immune system might be tricked by a dead virus, the result would be only short-term immunity. Enders and a University of Cincinnati researcher named Albert B. Sabin, the main opponents of rushing ahead with the Salk vaccine, were also concerned that a live virus might sneak through in a dead-virus batch and cause polio in someone who might not have gotten it otherwise.

While Sabin continued to work quietly on a live-virus vaccine, Salk was on the way to becoming a national hero, a veritable Lindbergh or Teddy Roosevelt. In 1954, nearly two million children took part in a study that inoculated some of them with the new vaccine and others with a placebo. In an indication of the naiveté of the times, many parents happily sent their children off to participate in an experiment that was undeniably dangerous.

But the experiment succeeded. As the vaccination program expanded, polio plummeted from a peak of 58,000 cases in 1952 to only 5,000 a few years later. Still, dissatisfaction with the killed-virus vaccine never did go completely away, and Sabin, ever Salk's nemesis, finally persuaded the government and the AMA that his vaccine was the better. With Sabin's vaccine—the one of choice for Western medicine, despite the continued use of Salk's in many places—polio has been defeated or is in retreat in most countries today, and the exaggerated terror it inspired is long past.

The advances against viruses continue. There is now a vaccine for the vicious hepatitis B virus, and vaccines for the potentially deadly influenza viruses. But herpes, another viral affliction, still flourishes, and the most ubiquitous of all the viral maladies—the common cold, caused by well over a hundred different viruses—may never be thwarted by a vaccine because the viruses are too numerous. And then there is AIDS, which in the early eighties appeared as a disease of unknown origin and unknown natural history for which there was no cure, no vaccine, and, initially, little that could be done to slow its progress or alleviate its symptoms. Rather quickly, medical scientists deduced that this devastating disease did its work not by causing a specific illness but by compromising the immune system itself and thus making the body vulnerable to a host of deadly ailments. AIDS now ranks among the most destructive plagues of the century, with millions infected worldwide by the beginning of the 1990s.

The first sign of the disease came in 1979 when the Centers for Disease Control in Atlanta spotted an unusually high incidence of a rare form of cancer, Kaposi's sarcoma, and a difficult-to-treat pneumonia among homosexual men. They soon noticed that the patients manifested sharp reductions in the white blood cells, or T-lymphocytes, that the body uses to fight off attack. As the disease

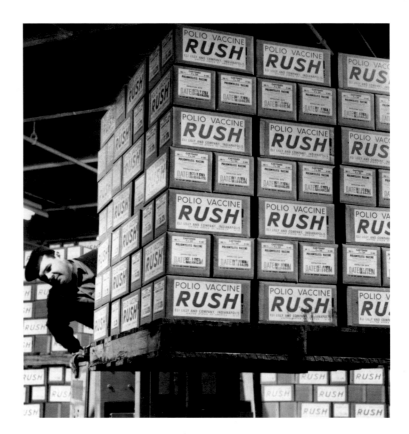

1955—(above) Finally, a polio vaccine—and the rush is on! Boxes of vaccine in an Indianapolis warehouse are kept under refrigeration to prevent spoilage. Photographed by Albert Fenn.

Circa 1950—(opposite) Polio epidemic, Hickory, North Carolina. Before the Salk and Sabin vaccines became available, children often received gamma globulin vaccinations. Photographed by Alfred Eisenstaedt.

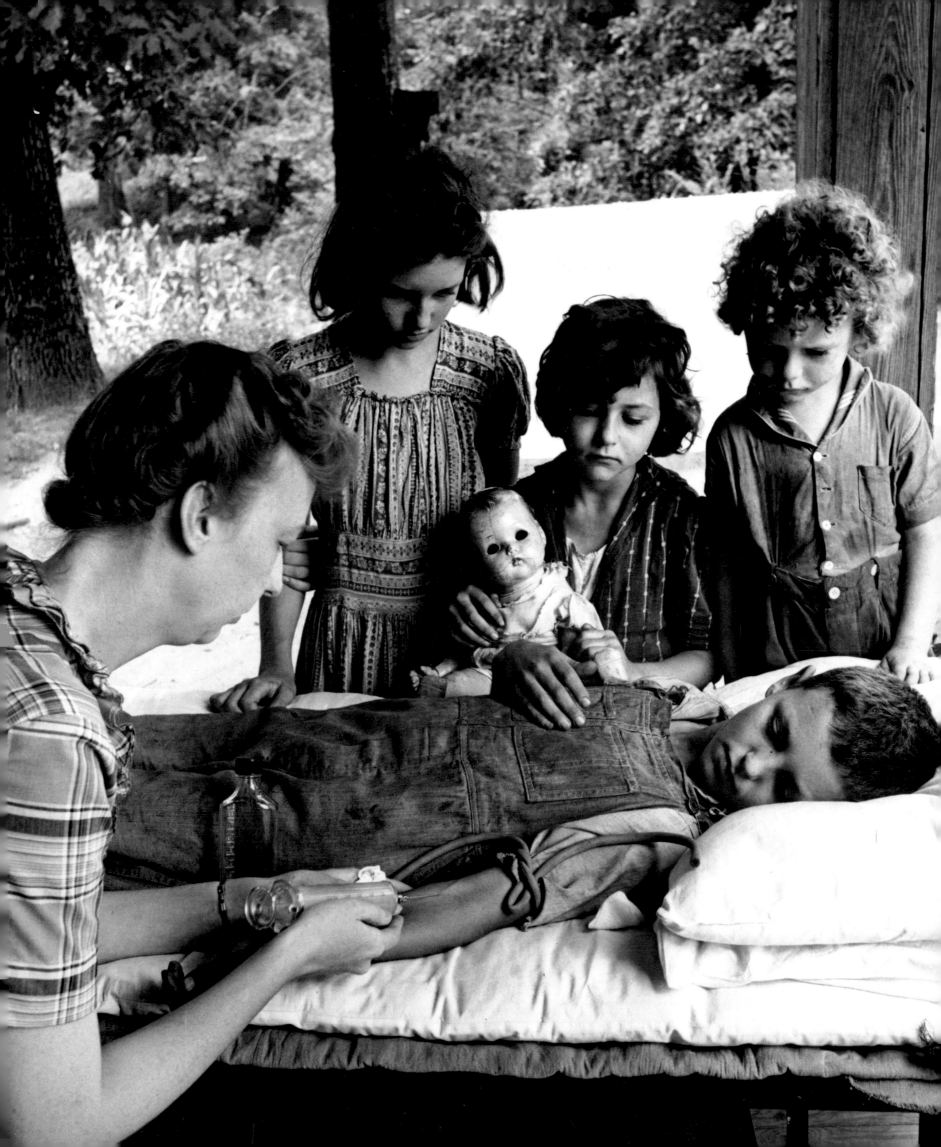

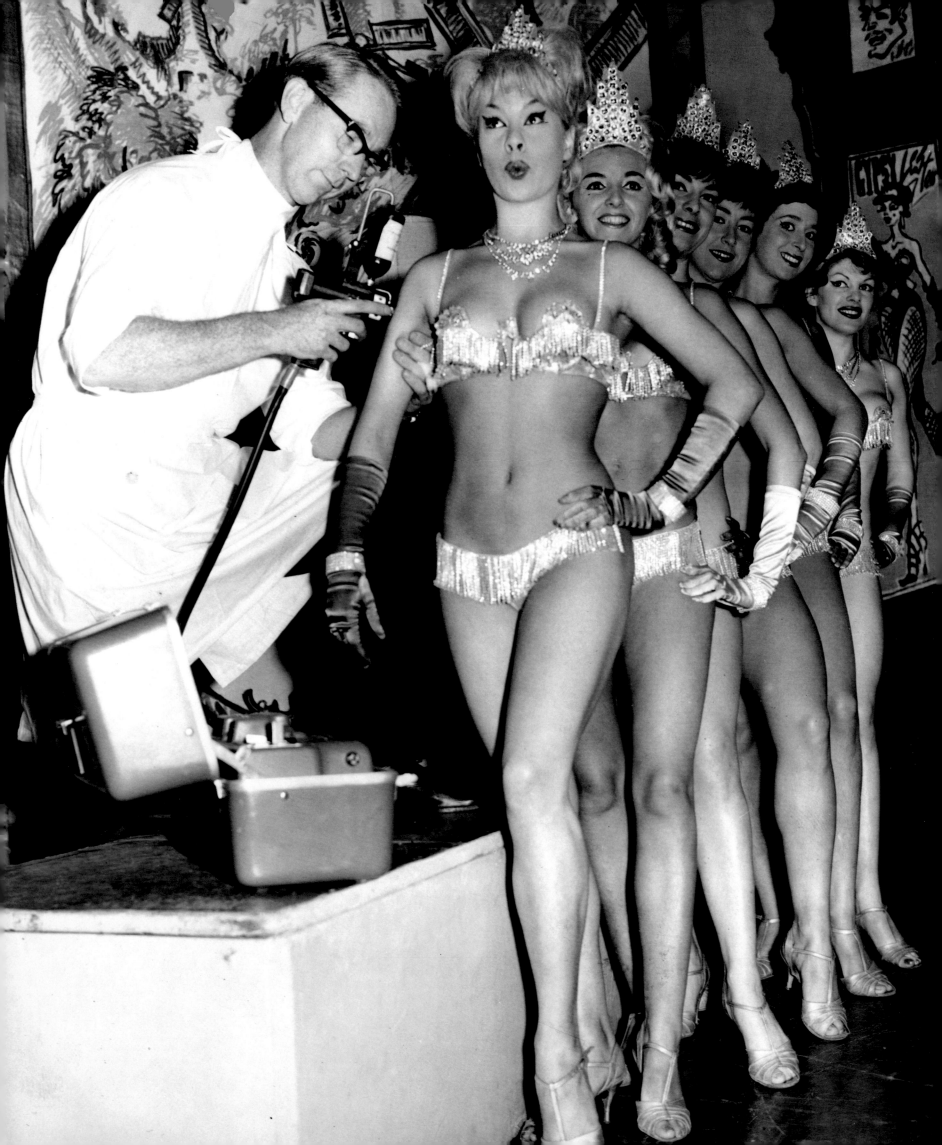

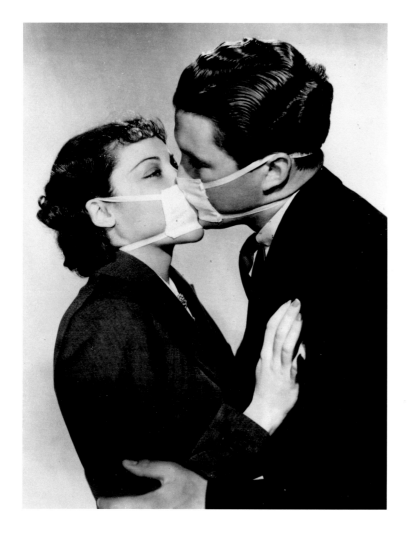

spread, so did a growing sense of panic. Fears that the blood supply might be contaminated proved justified. Heterosexuals, too, were shown to be vulnerable to the disease. Would medical science find nothing to defeat AIDS?

Considering the complexity of the situation, scientists were moving quite fast. In April 1984, Luc Montagnier, at the venerable Pasteur Institute in Paris, reported that he had found a virus he called LAV in eighty to ninety percent of the AIDS blood samples examined. At almost the same time, Dr. Robert Gallo of the National Institutes of Health in Bethesda asserted that the virus he had been studying, HTLV-III, looked like the culprit. As it turned out, they were both talking about the same virus, or at least similar strains of the same virus, and it would be called ultimately HIV, for Human Immunodeficiency Virus. The cause of this very difficult disease was isolated within five years after the new, mysterious disorder was first suspected. That it proved to be transmitted through the blood—by sexual activity, for instance, or the unclean needles of intravenous drug users—at least allowed for an educational campaign for safer sex and sterilization of needles.

Following this, the quest for a vaccine and for drugs that might cure AIDS accelerated. One medication, AZT (developed initially to fight cancer), was designated early on as a reasonably effective antiviral agent. Although it cannot eliminate the virus, AZT inhibits its spread from cell to cell and thus seems to prolong the lives of some AIDS sufferers. Other drugs remain, for the most part, promising but untested, or of limited value.

Just as AIDS underlines the frustrating knowledge that in medicine there is always something else around the corner, developments in both cancer and heart disease offer reason for optimism, though much work remains. George Nicholas Papanicolaou began reporting on his groundbreaking work on sex determination in guinea pigs as far back as 1917. These studies would lead, a quarter of a century

1963—(opposite) *London's Windmill Theater slogan: "We never close." And to make sure the show will, in fact, go on, Serena, Gina, Dawn, Doris, Pam, and Dierdre receive anti-influenza injections from a Crooks Laboratories team.*

Circa 1937—(above) *Hollywood, California. Hollywood was frightened. The flu could be as devastating to a production as a union strike. So during rehearsals, the actors (Betty Furness and Stanley Morner, better known by his stage name, Dennis Morgan) wore masks doused with an antiseptic and removed them only when the cameras began to roll. A physician named Harvey Washington Wiley promoted antiseptic kissing (Osculatio antiseptica) beyond the film set, but it never caught on.*

Circa 1940—(right) *Boy Scouts with signs, Louisville, Kentucky.*

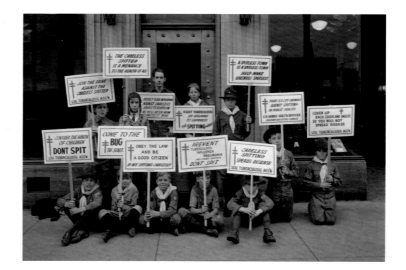

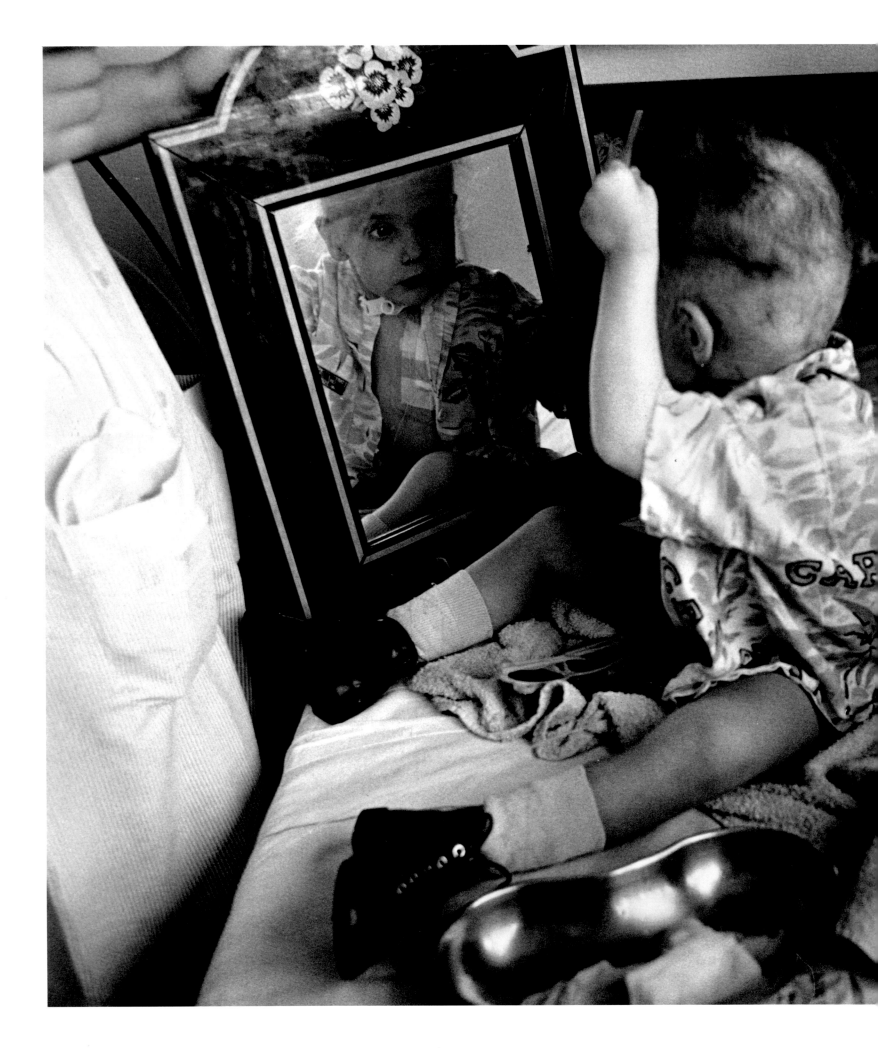

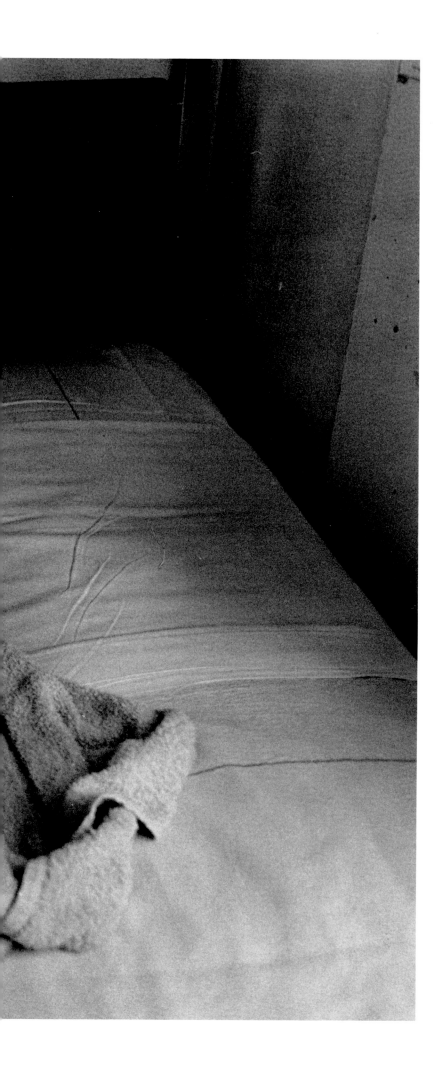

later, to the techniques for anticipating uterine tumors through a Pap smear, thus reducing the threat of uterine cancer. Early detection of all sorts of cancers has become a supreme weapon. Mammography is now accepted as safe and effective against breast cancer. Testicular cancer is curable when caught early, and colon cancer can be thwarted through routine examination. Skin cancer, spotted early, is almost routinely curable. Cancer has gone from being a disease that left medicine helpless to one for which the five-year survival rate for patients with major cancers today approaches fifty percent. (Nevertheless, cancer still strikes 1,130,000 Americans every year, killing many of them.)

If the capacity to detect cancer early and treat it has made dramatic strides, so has the capacity to prevent it. Although it is nearly impossible to stop some people from smoking—which causes eighty-five percent of cancers of the lung—no one can say medicine failed to warn them. The epidemiological triumph of the century began, for all practical purposes, in 1937. That was the year Professor Raymond Pearl of the Johns Hopkins School of Medicine published a paper in the journal *Science* in which he asserted, based on an analysis of biostatistics, that heavy smokers could expect to live less long than nonsmokers. Pearl's student E. Cuyler Hammond, joined by an associate, Daniel Horn, went on to develop a research project of mammoth proportions. Their study, begun in 1952, followed nearly 200,000 middle-aged men. By 1955, enough men had died in that group to allow a preliminary report. Final results in 1958 showed the association of smoking with the incidence of a wide spectrum of diseases. Heart disease was strikingly prominent. Besides lung cancer, there were cancers of the esophagus, larynx, pharynx, mouth, tongue, lip, and bladder. Laboratory tests that produced cancer in animals through direct manipulation of the smoking variable settled the case—despite tenacious resistance by the tobacco industry, a resistance that still persists, decades later.

While prevention and cure were advancing by great strides, there was also great frustration. Throughout the seventies and the eighties, scientists gradually told the story of cancer genes—genes that might be normal until they were activated by some trigger, perhaps by a carcinogen. If they had to be turned on to cause cancer, could there be a way of turning them off? As the decade ended, science seemed so close to the answers and yet so far.

For heart disease, the course of events has been similar. Just about one hundred years ago, in 1895, the renowned Viennese surgeon Theodor Billroth observed ominously: "No surgeon who wishes to preserve the respect of his colleagues would ever attempt to suture a

---

1989—*Child with cancer. In the last twenty to thirty years, remarkable strides have been made in childhood cancer, particularly the use of chemotherapy to combat leukemia. Photographed by J. L. Courtinat.*

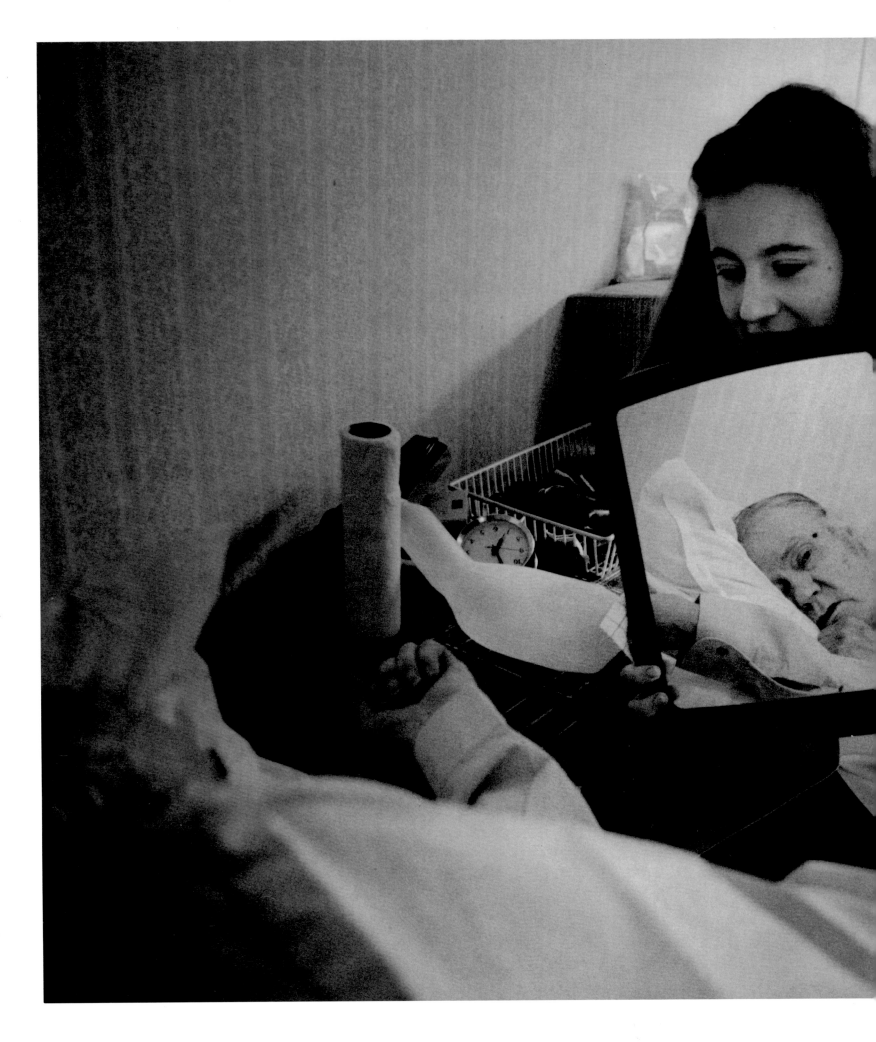

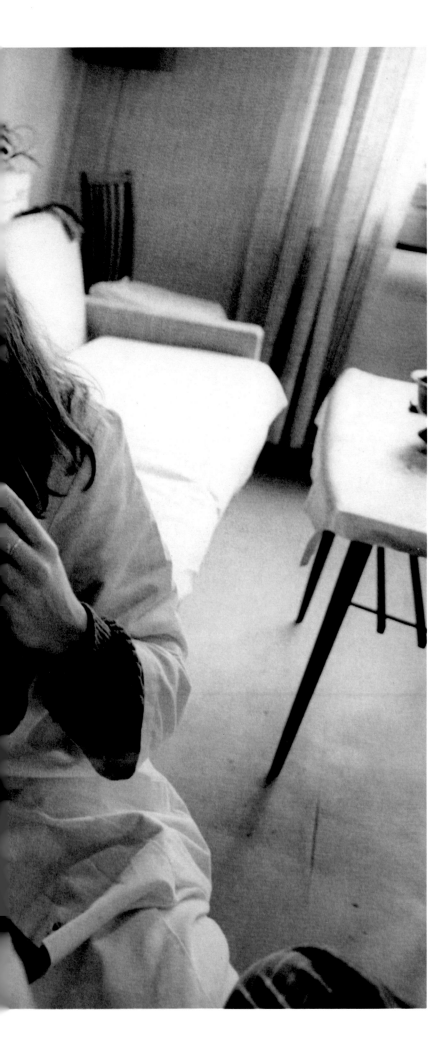

wound of the heart." There were, nonetheless, some heart operations in the first half of the century, perhaps most notably the 1945 operation developed by Dr. Helen B. Taussig and Dr. Alfred Blalock to correct the circulation blockage between lung and heart that created the infamous blue-baby syndrome.

But the biggest news was saved for the second half of the century. Open-heart surgery was a messy affair until the invention of the heart-lung machine by Dr. John H. Gibbons, Jr., in 1953 freed up the organs while blood was being oxygenated mechanically outside the body during surgery. This, in turn, made possible the most startling heart development of the century when, in 1967, Dr. Christiaan Barnard, a South African surgeon, performed the first transplantation of the heart of one human into the chest of another. By the late 1980s there were thousands of people throughout the world living with someone else's heart. One illustrious example, Emmanuel Vitria of Marseilles, France, survived for over eighteen years after his 1969 transplant, dying at the age of sixty-seven.

As the heart transplant became more practical, a new concern arose. There were just not enough hearts to go around. This led to experiments like the Jarvik 7, a machine designed to replace a patient's heart permanantly. Though unsuccessful, attempts to create artificial hearts showed that false optimism had got the upper hand. It really is no wonder, since so many medical miracles had occured in so short a time. But progress continued. The relationship of diet to heart disease was clear, especially as reflected in blood levels of cholesterol, resulting in a revolution in the way many people regard food. Angioplasty, developed in 1977 by Dr. Andreas Gruentizig in Zurich, cleared a passage through clogged coronary arteries by inflating a ballon into the space. Drugs called beta blockers—used earlier in Europe and then approved in the United States in 1967—proved that blood pressure could be lowered, blood vessels dilated, and the heart's work made easier, thus preventing subsequent heart attacks. A laser-beam device came along to vaporize arterial obstructions. Techniques were developed to replace faulty heart valves. Coronary bypasses to replace diseased arteries with healthy ones became commonplace; more than 125,000 bypasses were being performed yearly in the 1980s.

No matter how effective medicine's tools of drugs and technology have become, the heart's power of life and death has the last word, and remedying the twentieth-century phenomenon of heart disease ultimately means changing behavior and values, which is medicine's strongly worded message to the public today.

———————

1990—*Home for the aged in Sweden.*
Photographed by Anders Petersen.

1990—*(Following page) Baby with AIDS, Romania.*
Photographed by Bernard Bisson.

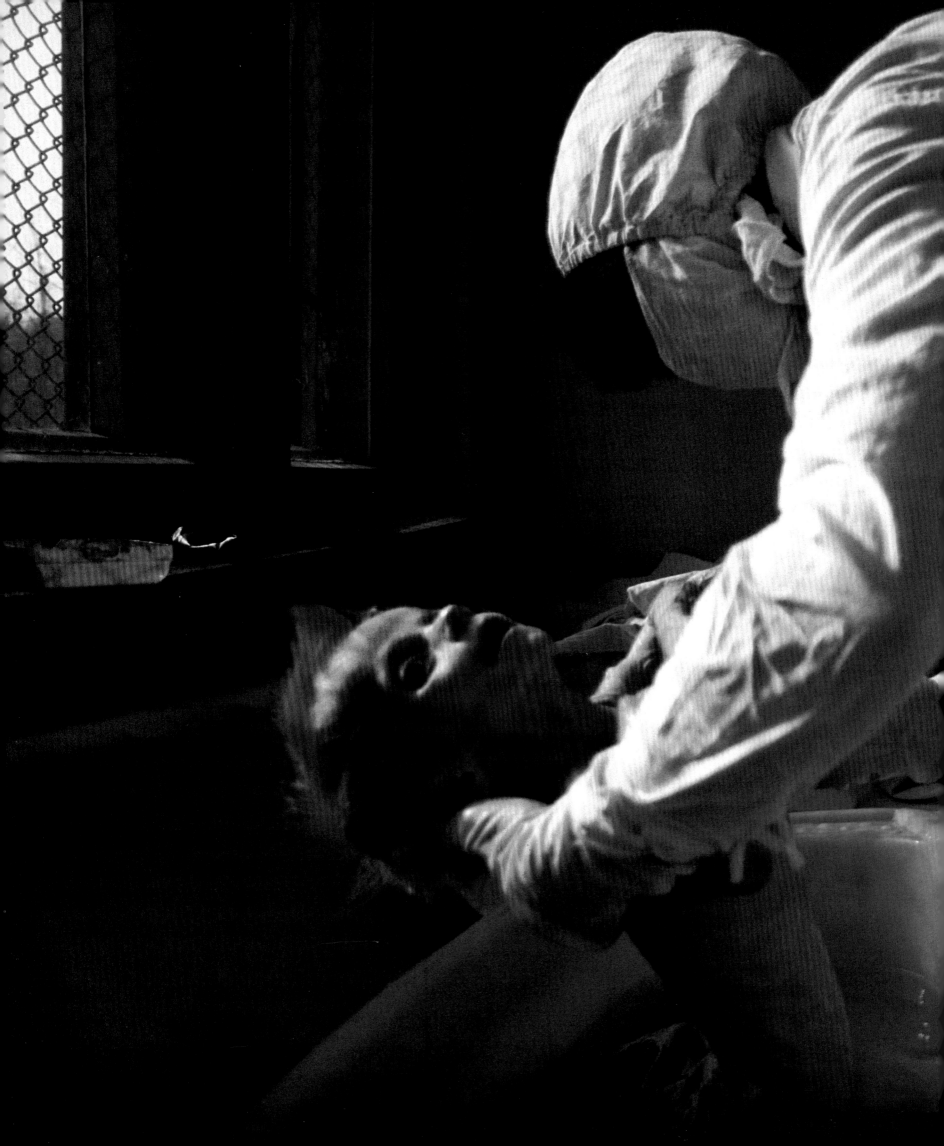

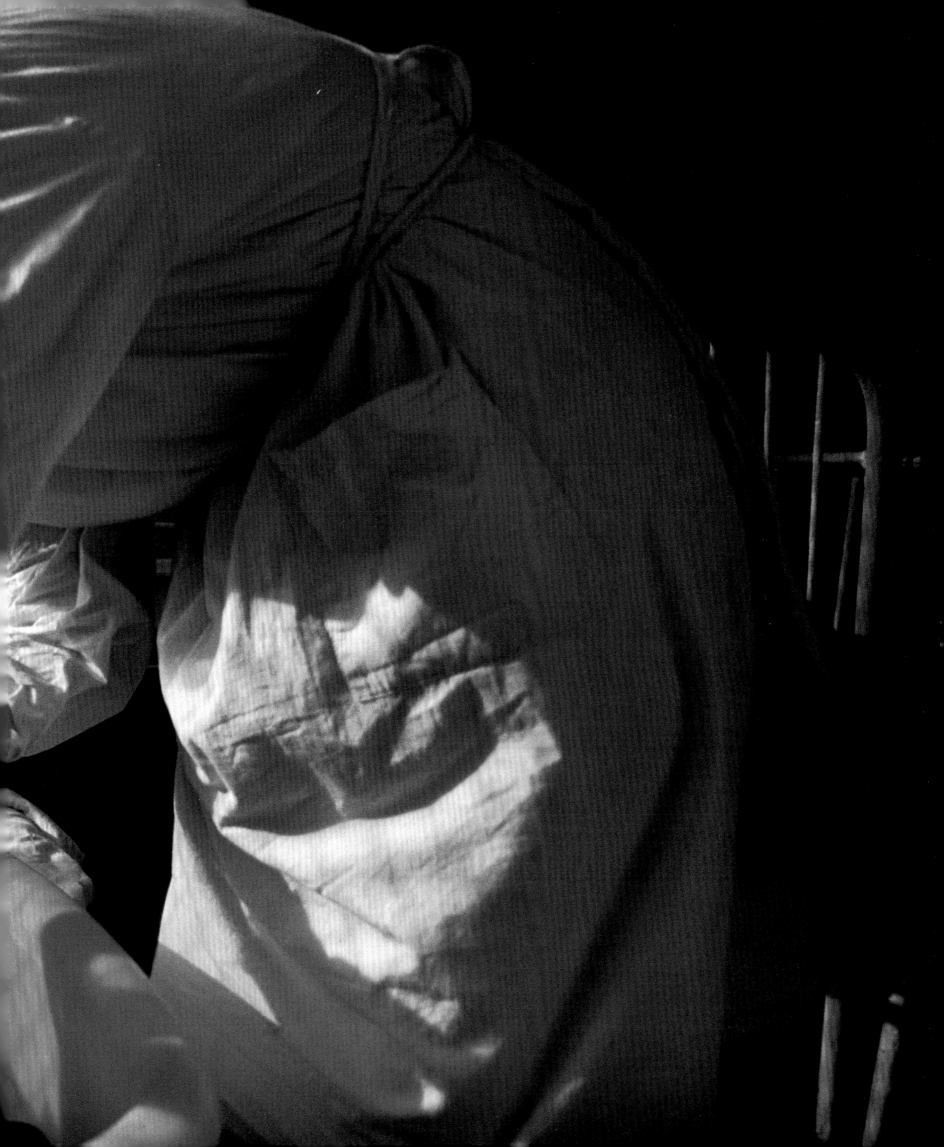

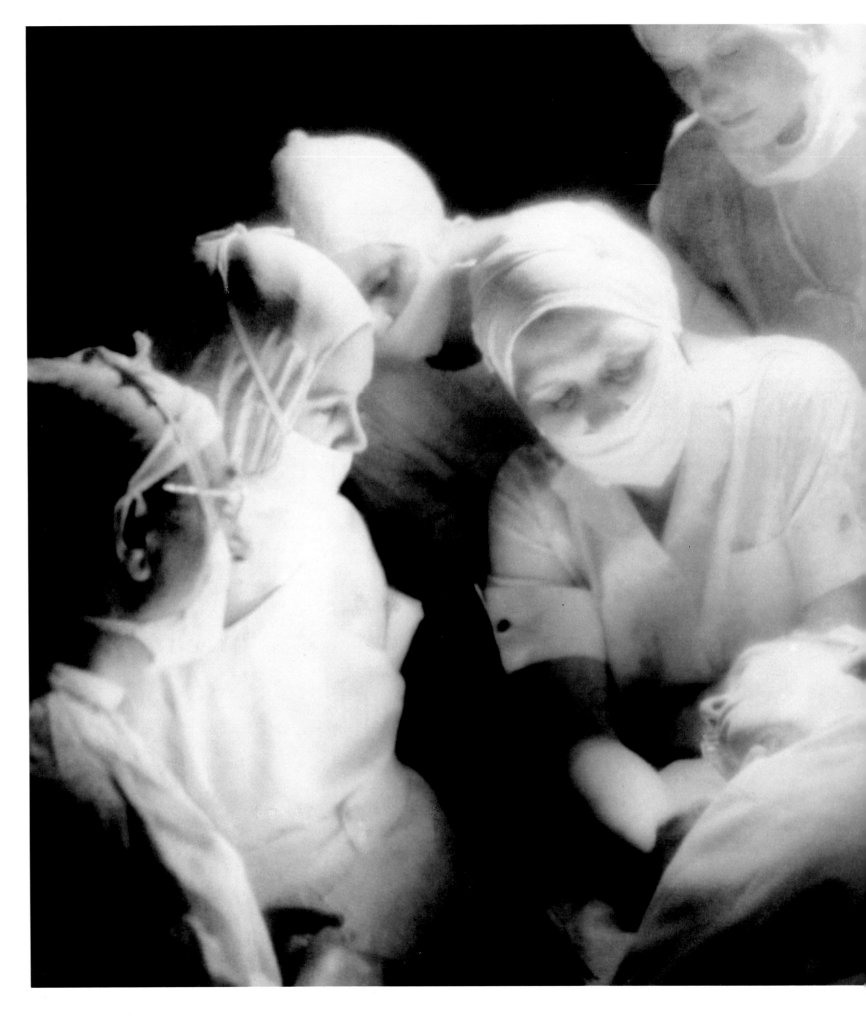

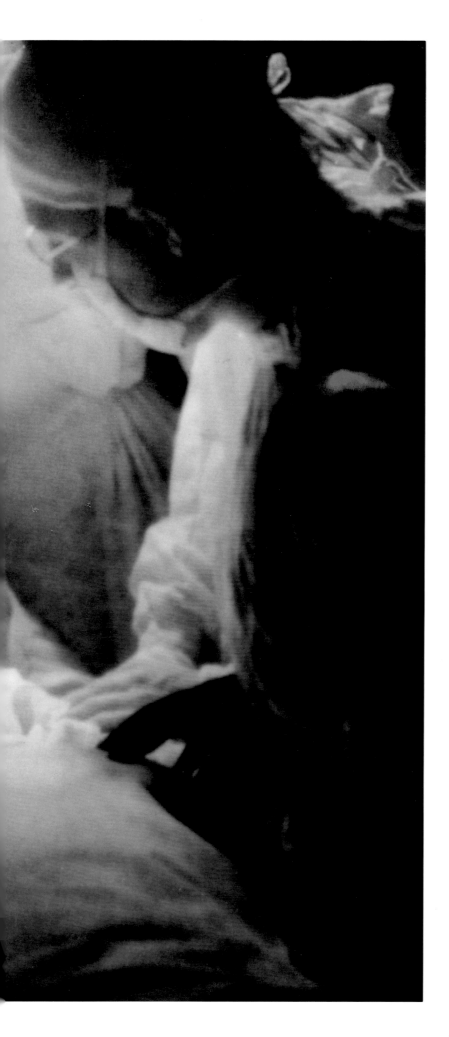

CHAPTER TWO

A GROWING TRUST

THE TWENTIETH CENTURY WAS ONE OF NEWFOUND CONFI-
DENCE: AFTER SO MANY YEARS MARKED BY EMPTY POSTURING
AND FALSE PROMISES, MEDICINE FINALLY HAD GENUINE HELP
TO OFFER, THANKS TO BETTER TRAINING OF DOCTORS, SO-
PHISTICATED SURGERY, AND THE DEVELOPMENT OF MODERN
HOSPITALS. ONCE-WARY PATIENTS WERE NOW WILLING TO
TRUST THEIR DOCTORS WITH THEIR LIVES INSIDE A VISION OF
ORDER THAT THE WELL-SCRUBBED WARDS AND THE GLEAM-
ING AMPHITHEATERS OF THE HOSPITAL PROVIDED.

Today, many of us choose to fight illness at home—but only as
long as the malady seems minor. At the first sign of any real risk,
sometimes sooner, we head for the hospital. Yet the hospital itself is
essentially a twentieth-century phenomenon. In 1800 there were
only two hospitals in all of America: New York Hospital, founded
in 1771, and Pennsylvania Hospital in Philadelphia, founded in
1751. By 1909 there were 4,359 hospitals; by 1992, 6,649 were in
existence. As the twentieth century moved along, house calls faded
from common experience and the doctor's office and clinics took
over almost entirely for out-patient medical care, becoming more
and more like mini-hospitals, with nurses and diagnostic machinery. Many doctors' offices and clinics retained only the semblance of
noninstitutional practice, situated as they were in the vicinity of a
hospital so that office and hospital could work in tandem.

Watching this evolution, many observers expressed alarm
over the loss of the personal touch. They saw an estrangement of
patient and doctor, as medicine increasingly turned to teams,
technology, and high-powered institutions. Others welcomed the
inevitable, seeing an overall increase in quality and efficiency. This

*1935—The photographer Max Thorek depicted tension in the operating
room in an image he called* Suspense. *While dramatic advances were made
in all health care fields in the twentieth century, progress was nowhere more
pronounced than in surgery.*

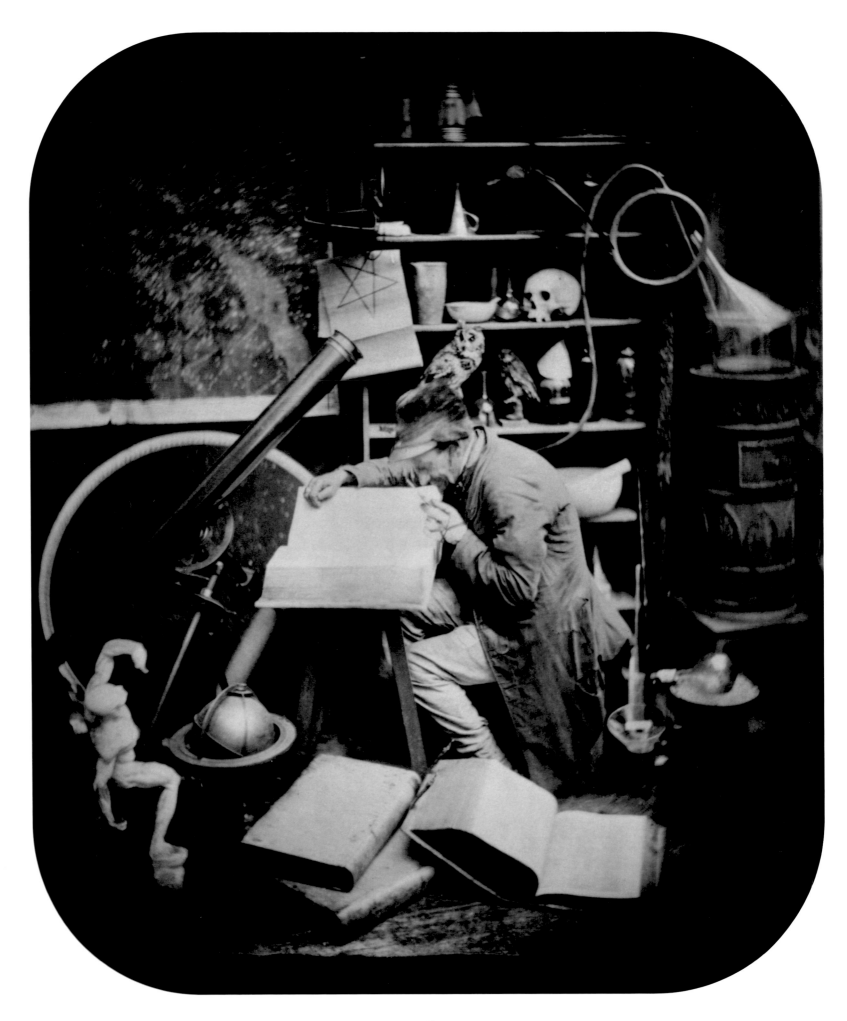

Circa 1853—*(opposite) Despite some significant strides, medical care in the nineteenth century was often undermined by occult practices and sheer quackery. This early daguerrotype depicts the sort of self-styled doctor who gave scientific medicine a bad reputation.*

Circa 1860—*(right) Bloodletting, the process of bleeding a patient, was a popular medical technique. The operation was divided into two categories: general, which consisted of opening a vein (venisection) or an artery (arteriotomy), and local, which involved cupping or leeching (sanguisuction). Sometimes, bloodletting was done routinely in the spring as a prevention against disease. It was assumed that women, who bled naturally each month, could especially benefit from an additional loss of blood. In 1835, French physician Pierre-Charles-Alexandre Louis employed the new techniques of medical statistics to analyze the procedure and decided that bloodletting was useless. But the practice was slow to die. In this English* carte de visite, *the doctor uses a steel instument tipped with sharp blades to minister to his patient.*

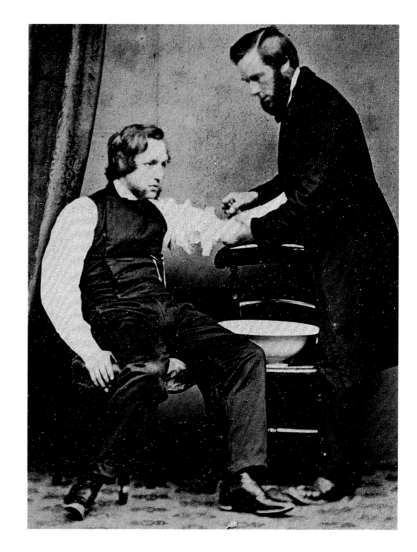

transition did not happen suddenly. As the earliest technology emerged, doctors realized they needed some hospital affiliation for access to the machinery and the accumulated expertise there. The community hospitals, to take one vibrant example, were born to satisfy that need. They gave local physicians a way to intertwine their practices with the resources of a neighborhood institution. But even many of these small, intimate places saw explosive growth around the turn of the century. The modest Watts Hospital in Durham, North Carolina, described itself in 1895 as a "cottage hospital." Twenty-five years and a one-million-dollar endowment later, Watts boasted a pathology department and an X-ray department, and it was performing over 1,500 operations a year.

As the modern hospital evolved—particularly the major institution with ties to a university—surgery, modern medicine, and education all came to reside in a single temple of health. Bigness would come to matter, not only because of the technical and teaching resources a large hospital might provide, but also because of the prestige that went along with the accumulation of a critical mass of high-quality people. A great deal had to precede this full emergence of the multifaceted, respected hospital of modern times.

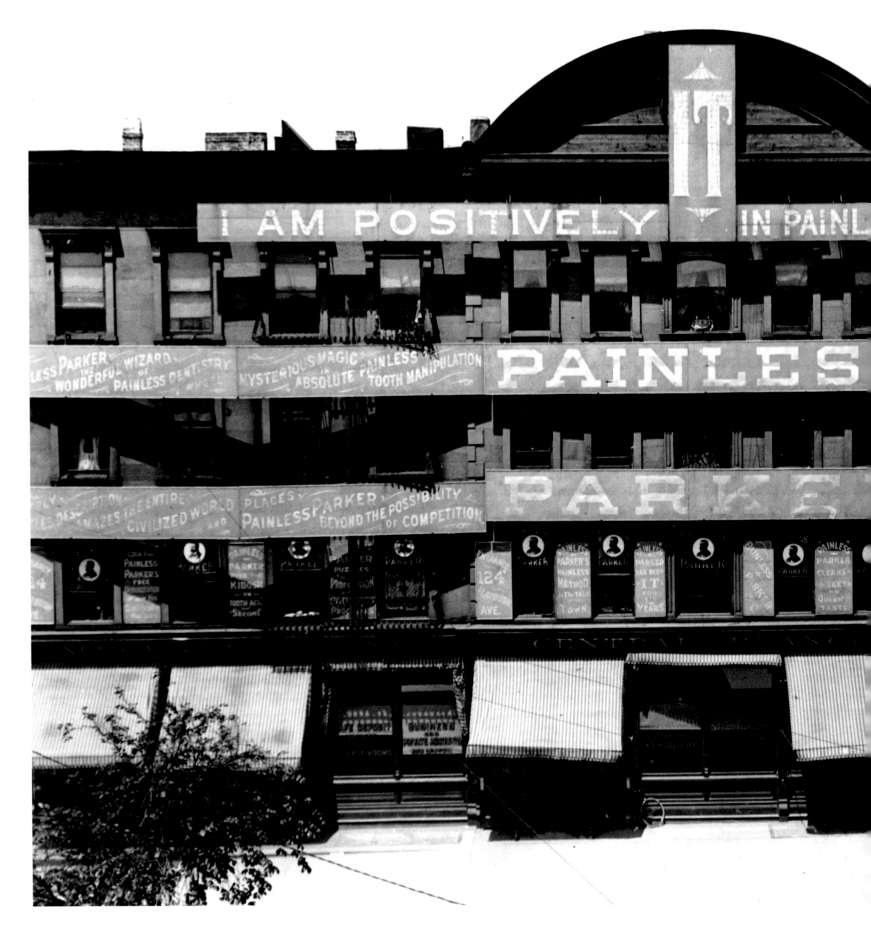

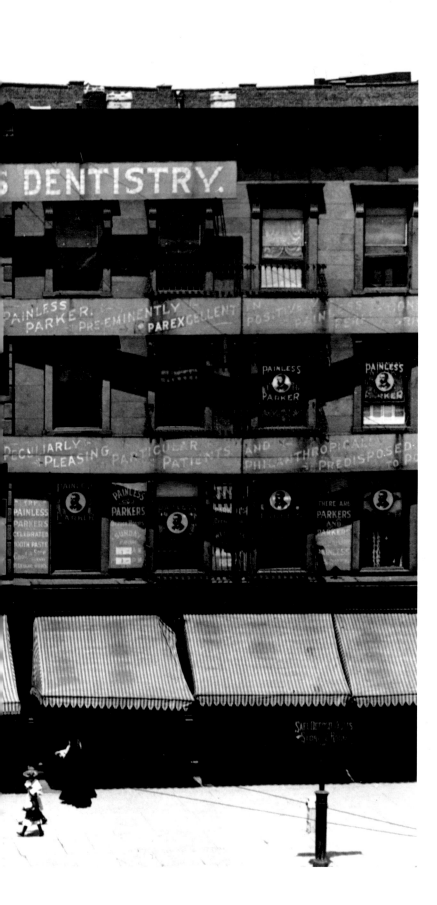

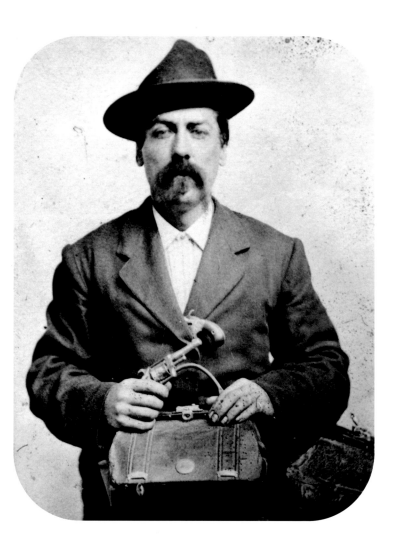

Circa 1930—*(left) Painless Parker Dental Parlors flourished in New York City in the late 1920s and 1930s. The sign on this building on Flatbush Avenue in Brooklyn extends nearly a full block.*

Circa 1884—*(above) In the line of duty, Alfred Harrison Neal, or "Doc Neal," an Ozark physician, ran into big trouble on a house call. He was fatally shot in the back by one Ice Sturgeon in 1889, after Doc accused Ice of having an affair with his wife.*

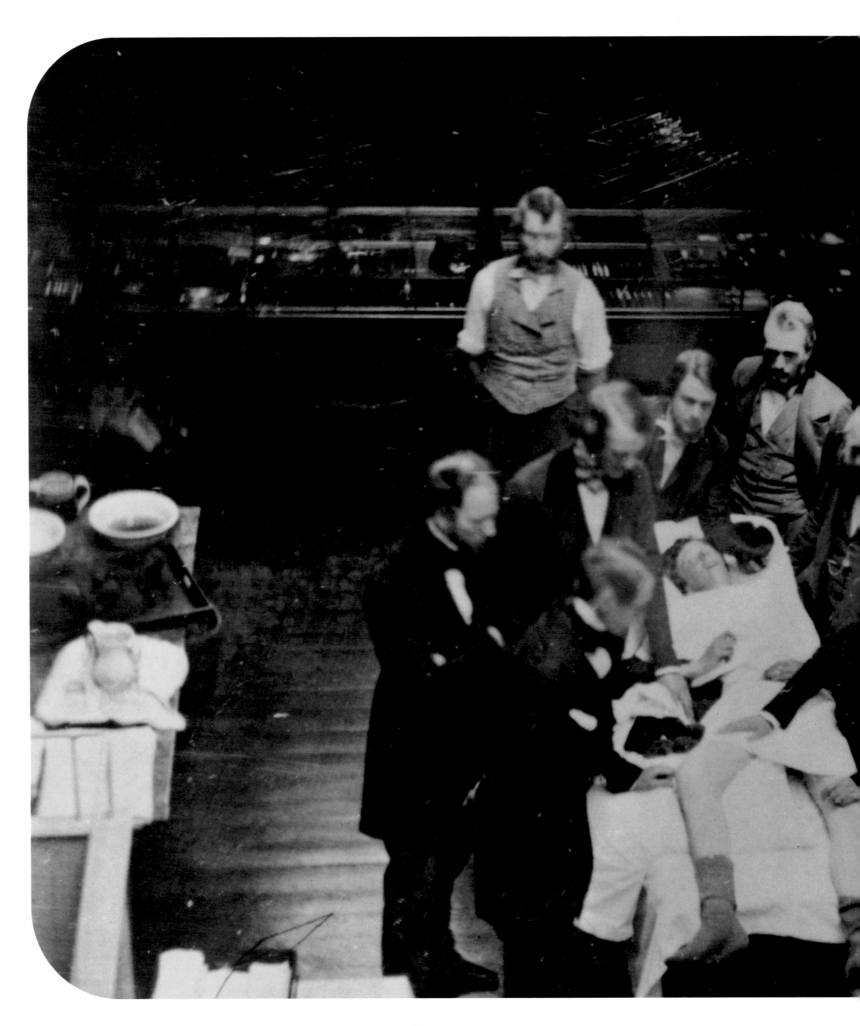

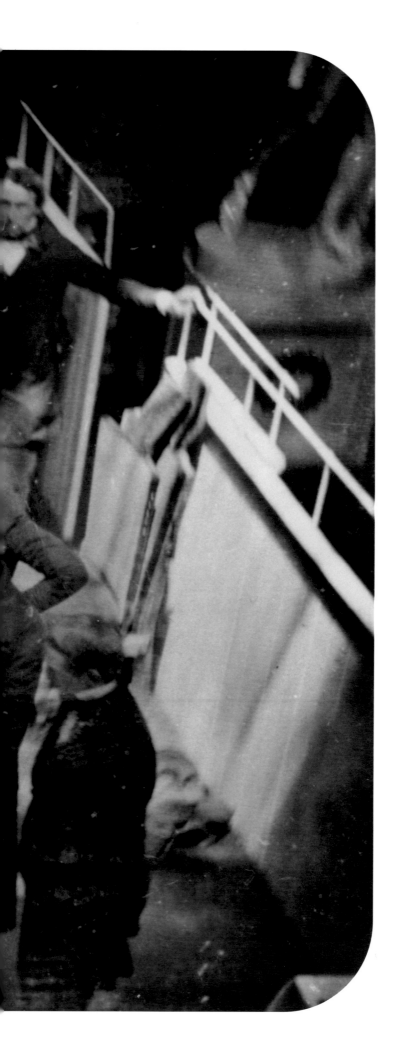

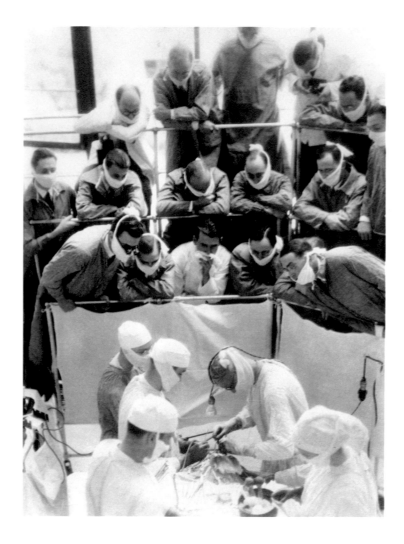

Surgery played a central role. In the nineteenth century, an operation was a bleak, brutal business. A surgeon virtually had to be an athlete, calling on all his dexterity and strength. In light of the unavoidable and excruciating pain involved, he had to get in, get out, and then hope for the best. Obviously, only the simplest of operations could be widely performed: amputations, the repair of gunshot wounds, the treatment of fractures. The procedures were fast; even so, in the middle of the nineteenth century, Valentine Mott, a New York surgeon, wrote of "individuals praying in mercy

---

Circa 1848—(left) Anesthesia was first used in 1846, in a pioneering operation at Massachusetts General Hospital. Its advent opened the way for many startling advances in twentieth-century medicine. The man with his hand on the patient's thigh is John Collins Warren, co-founder of the hospital; across from him is Oliver Wendell Holmes, the eminent author and physician whose son became a Supreme Court Justice. Photographed by Southworth and J. J. Hawes.

1932—(above) After anesthesia, cleanliness was the other great innovation in surgery. The revered surgeon Harvey Cushing is pictured with a group of fellow doctors in surgical masks during an operation at the Peter Bent Brigham Hospital which introduced many precautions against infection.

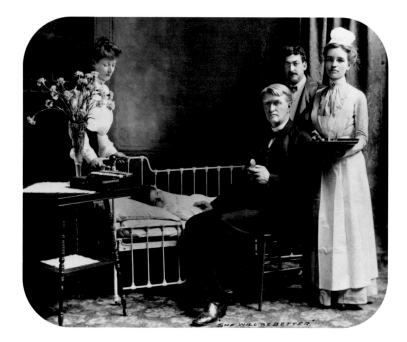

that we would stop, that we would finish, thus imploring and menacing us, and those patients would not fail to escape if they were not firmly secured."

Under these circumstances, ether was a gift from heaven. Anesthetic agents had been known for a long time but were not extensively used in surgery until the 1840s, first in Britain and France and then in the United States. Even so, the practice of surgery did not change radically. The reason was that people too often died from the operation anyway. Painless or not, surgery still tended to be fatal because infection, rather than healing, was the usual outcome. In fact, ether and chloroform, by permitting more lengthy, invasive operations, allowed for even greater chance of infection. And the hospital was certainly no place to go willingly for any procedure. People got sick there, often dying of an illness contemporary wags called "hospitalism."

Just as hospitals needed the surgery business to energize them, the advancement of surgery awaited the development of safer hospitals—an eventuality that would not occur until the twentieth century, although throughout the nineteenth the efforts to purify hospitals were strenuous enough. Even though Pasteur and then Lister were doing the work that would solidify germ theory as an explanation for infection, the prevailing idea of infection in the 1800s was a much less precise one, involving poisons in the air that needed to be diluted with fresh breezes. Even the legendary Florence

---

Circa 1900—*(above) Separate facilities for children in general hospitals began around the turn of the century. Independent hospitals for children began to appear in the 1870s. Photographed by W. H. Willard Jones.*

Circa 1890—*(right) Patient with nurse at the Hôpital Saint-Louis, Paris.*

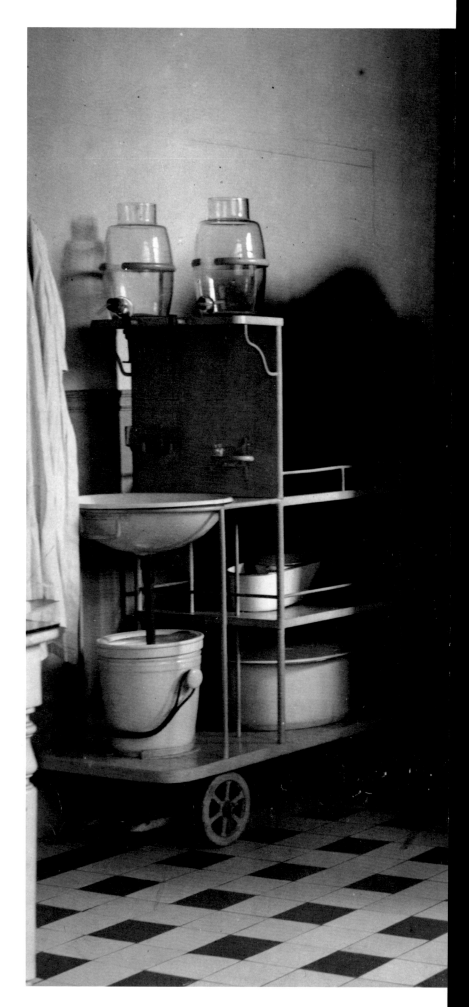

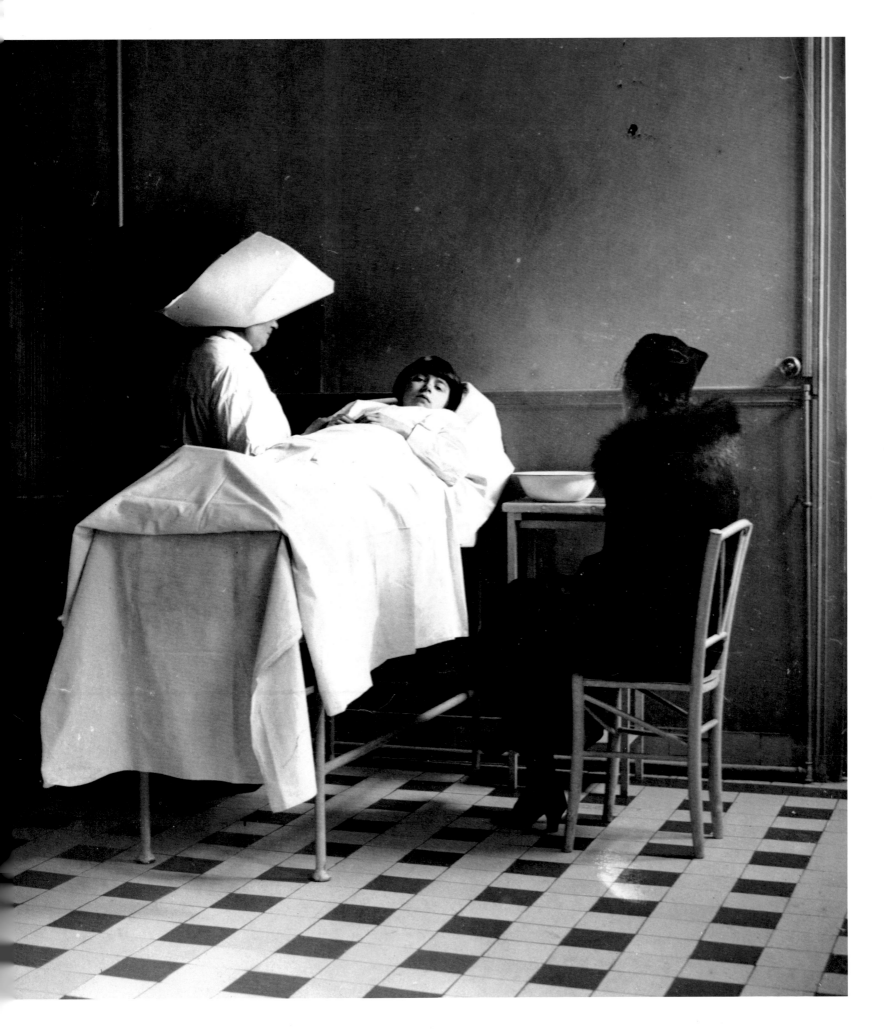

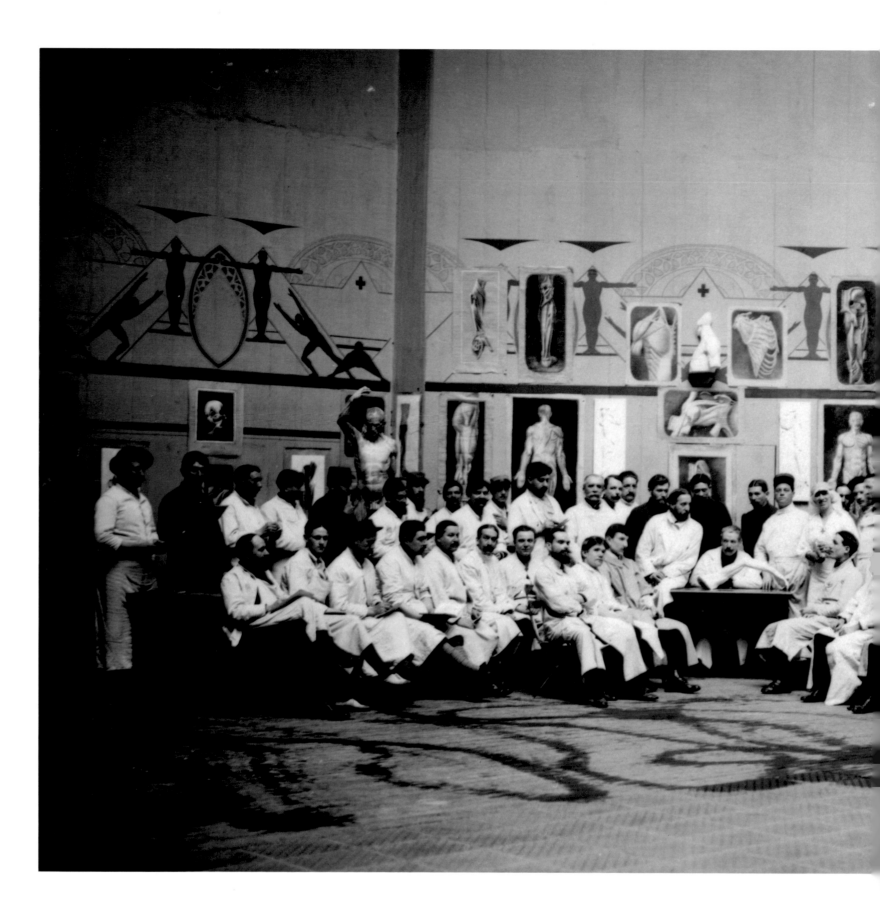

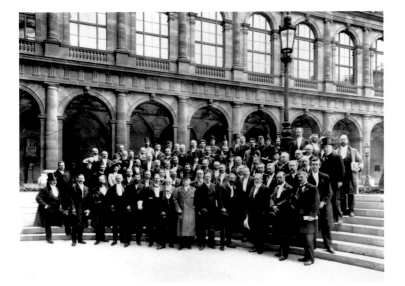

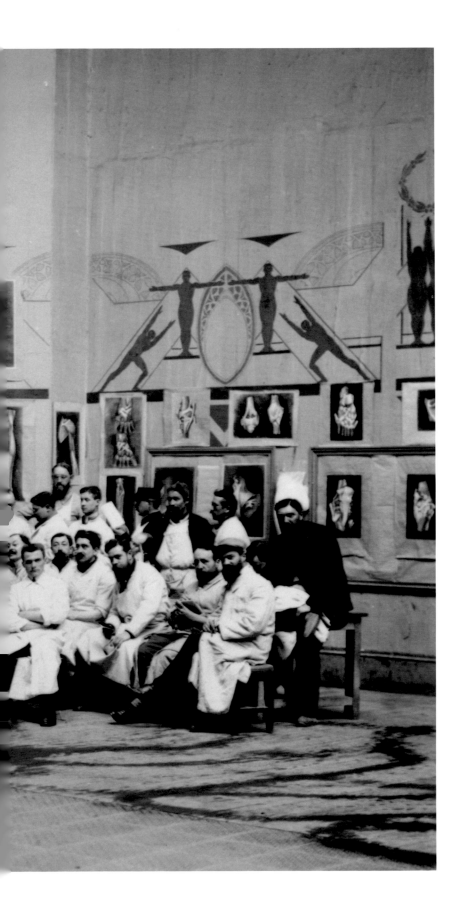

Nightingale, pushing for hospital reform and for rigorous sanitation, believed the atmosphere caused disease. The hospital became a moral battleground in which the dirty did battle with the clean. To be sanitary, a hospital had to have plenty of windows open to a constant breeze and to be far from the contagions thought to be carried by crowds.

THE SEAT OF INFLUENCE

In the decades before this century, the center of Western medicine was not New York or Massachusetts but rather Germany and Austria. There, the greatest laboratory advances were being made, and the teaching of doctors had been revolutionized and tied to those laboratory advances. Medicine was gradually assuming the mantle of science instead of the aura of superstition and guesswork. Americans were by comparison and even by their own estimation mired in a backwater. According to medical historian Thomas Bonner, half the leading U.S. doctors born between 1850 and 1890 studied in Germany, while Vienna alone drew some ten thousand American physician-trainees between 1870 and 1914. But during that very same period, the United States was positioning itself to seize the lead in modern medicine and surgery. Soon (and this must have seemed almost incredible to European surgical luminaries like Theodor Billroth) North America would become the mecca for the world's physicians.

The story of how this explosive expansion in science and skill was achieved has many subplots. But nearly all emphasize the

1920—(left) Military hospital, Grand Palais, Paris.

1907—(above) Early in the century, medicine was clearly taking on the trappings and the posture of a fraternity: the gathered physicians at the International Tuberculosis Conference, Vienna.

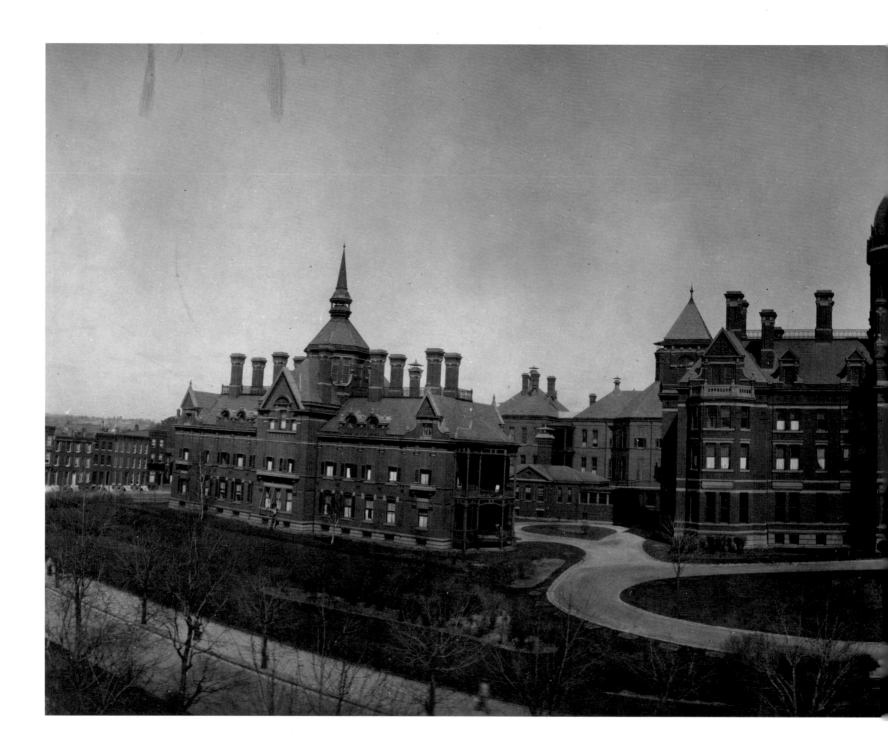

contributions of a remarkable phalanx of physicians working together at Johns Hopkins University. There, what was known as the
German system of medical training would take hold, flourish, and
reach out to other regions. In the story of Hopkins, the work and
influence of William Halsted—unquestionably among the greatest
surgeons ever born—is preeminent. In the annals of medicine, he
may have no parallel. Yet he was a tragic figure, too, whose bold
experiments with drugs led to his addiction.

Halsted started out as something of a dilettante, a Yale
athlete who appeared to lack the intellectual discipline that distinguished scholarship required. Dabbling early on *(continued on page 75)*

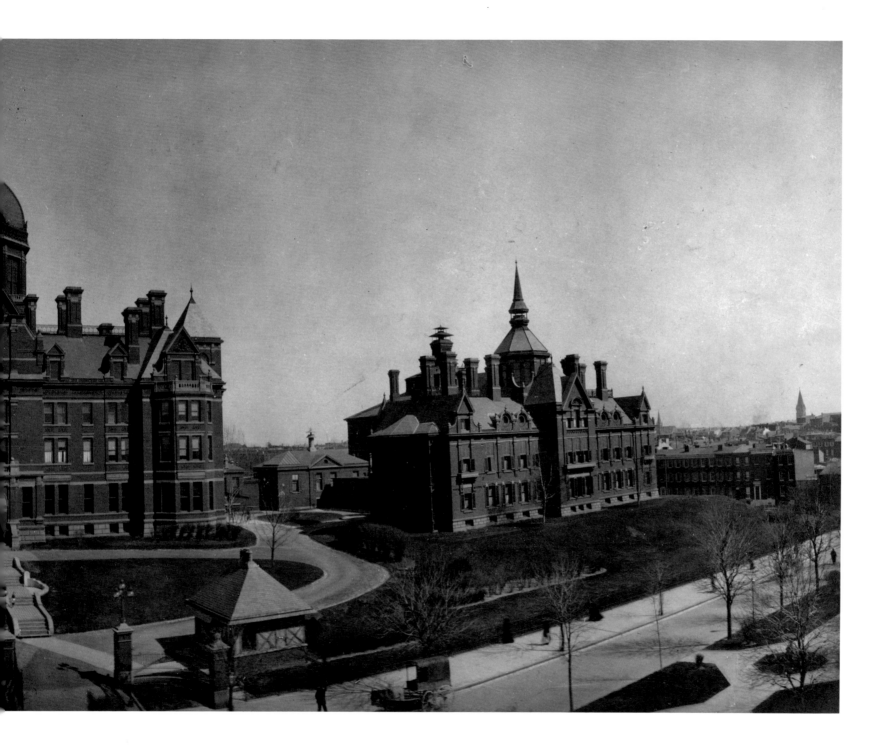

Circa 1890—*There were already other eminent hospitals in the United States, but Johns Hopkins Hospital in Baltimore, which opened in 1889, quickly leapt to the forefront. Working closely with its medical school, it became a pioneering teaching hospital, thanks in large measure to its distinguished staff. The hospital brought together William Osler, William S. Halsted, William H. Welch, and Howard A. Kelly, all of whom helped to draw the attention of the world's medical community to the United States and to scientific medicine.*

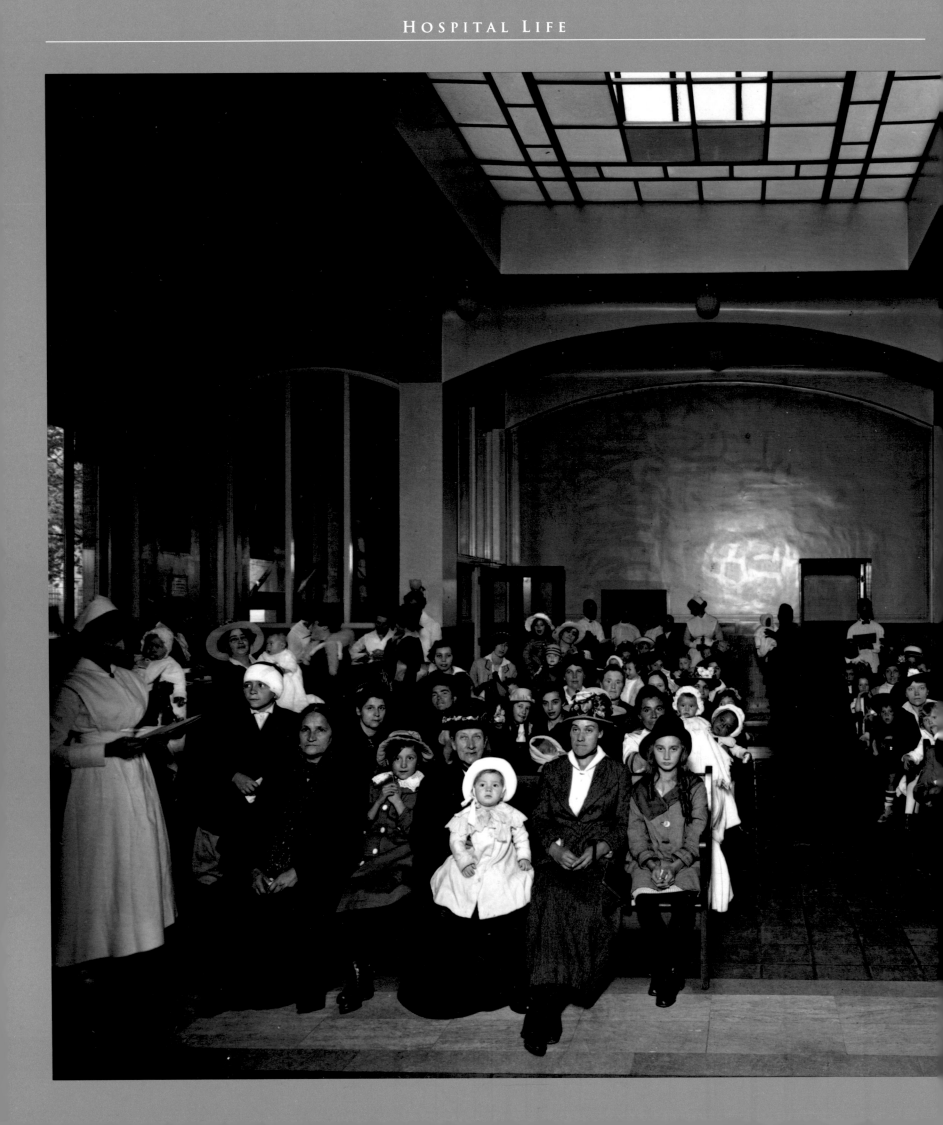

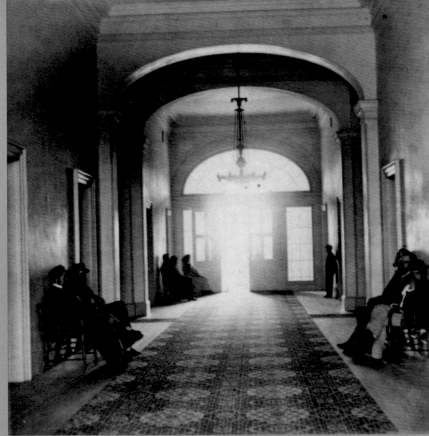

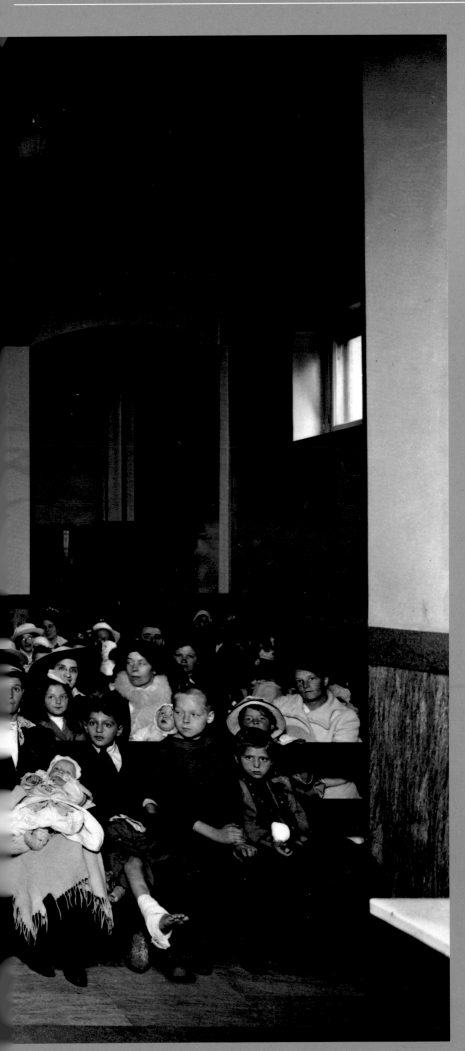

Hospital Life —
100 Years Ago

Circa 1910—*(left)* Endowed with greater resources and prestige, hospitals were founded in growing numbers as the twentieth century progressed. Hospitals gradually lost their forbidding aura and medical care was extended to ever more people, as can be seen in the crowded waiting room of Toronto's Hospital for Sick Children.

Circa 1915—*(above)* A crusade to bring brightness and ventilation to every new institution transformed the appearance of hospitals. The medical world now believed that light and air were key elements of health. (What a contrast to the somber almshouses of the past!) The waiting room for men at the Pennsylvania Hospital reflects the airiness of new hospital design.

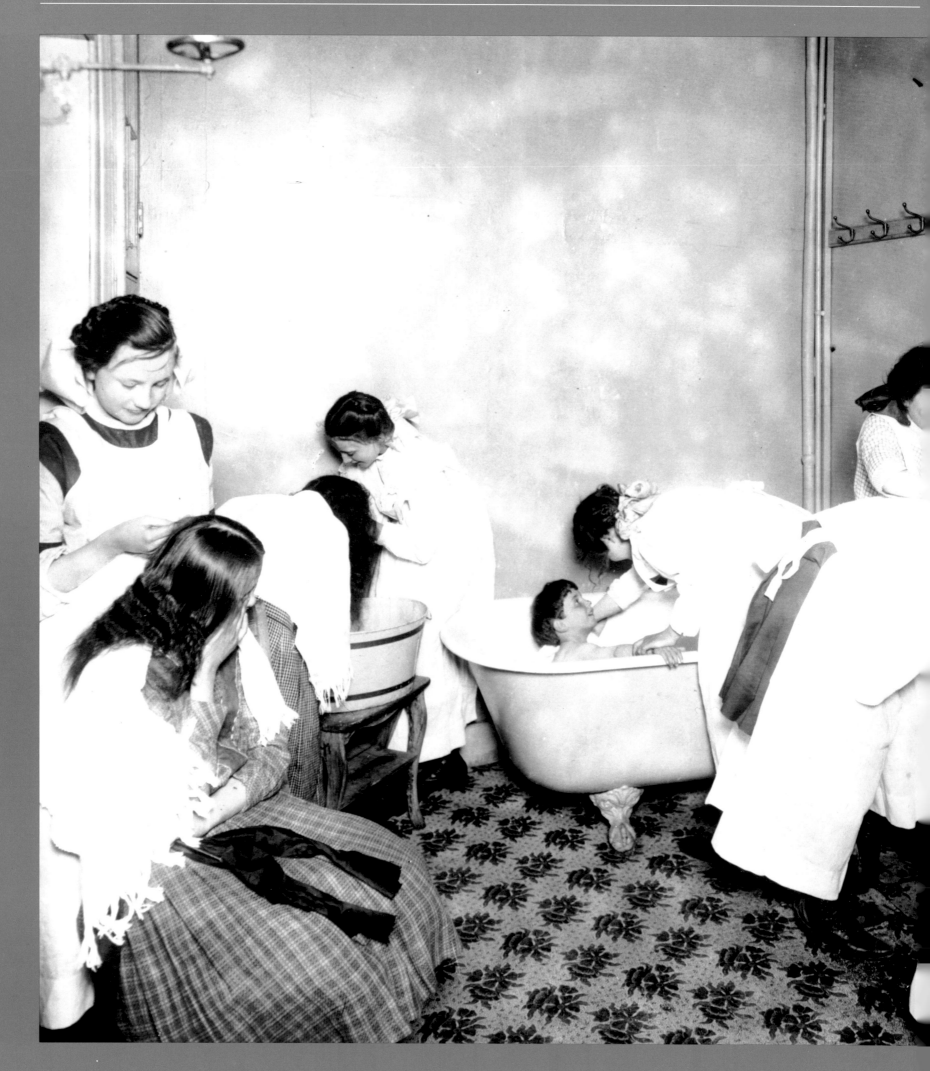

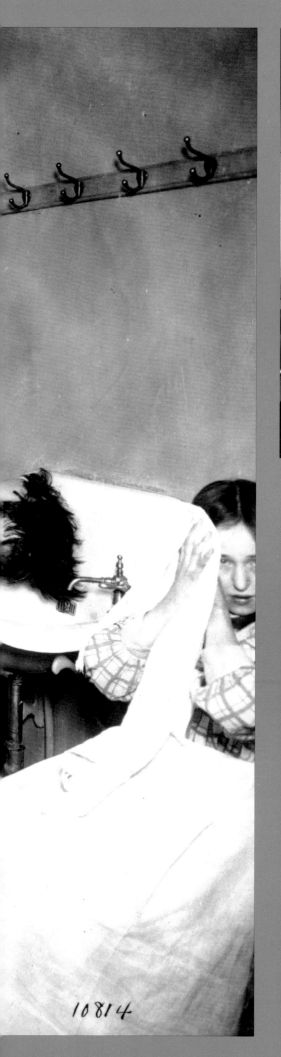

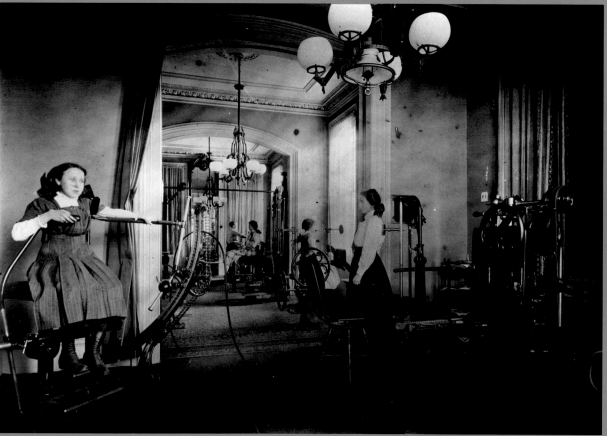

Circa 1920—*(left)* In many ways the early twentieth-century hospital was becoming an extension of the family, fostering personal care that was not necessarily designed to cure a specific illness. It had become an educational institution, or a temple perhaps, nurturing reverence for the new values of sanitation and physical well-being. At New York's Bellevue Hospital, as seen here, the nurses conduct a girls' class in personal cleanliness.

Circa 1915—*(above)* At the New Haven Hospital in Connecticut, newfangled physical therapy machines are put to use amid elegant surroundings.

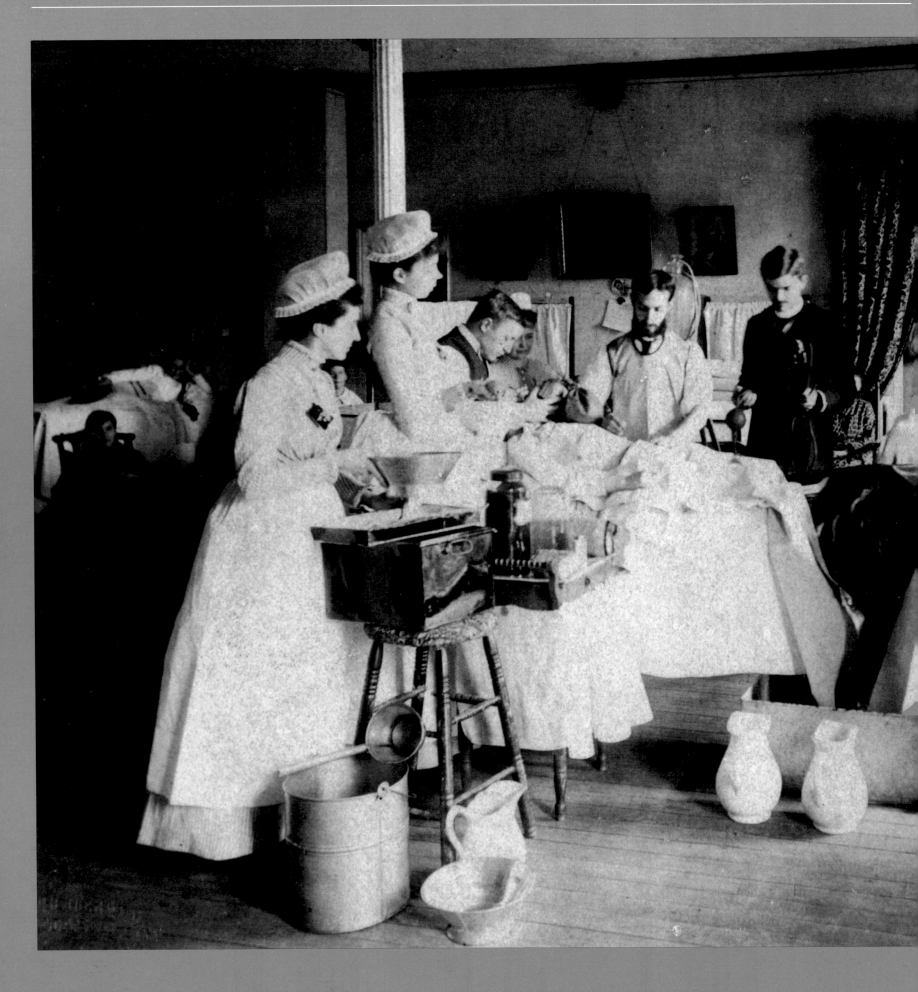

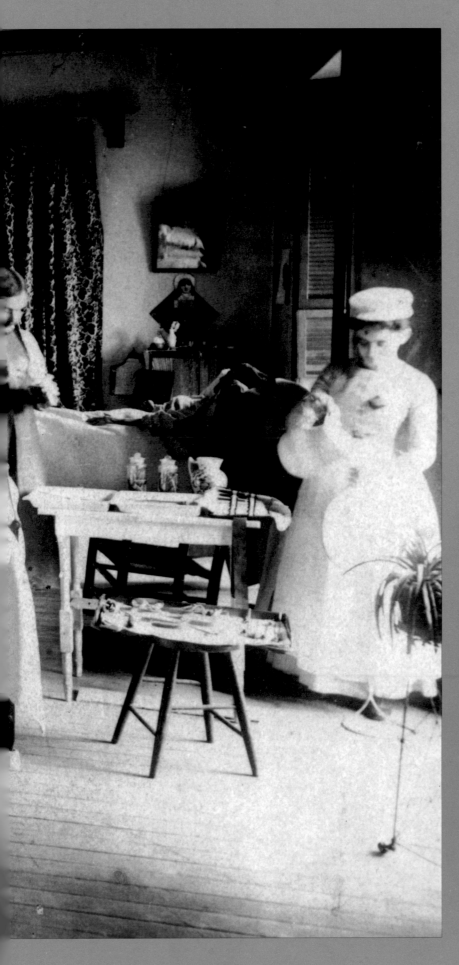

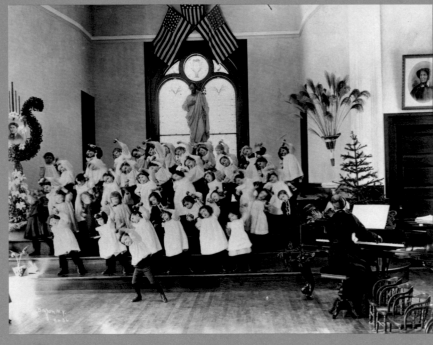

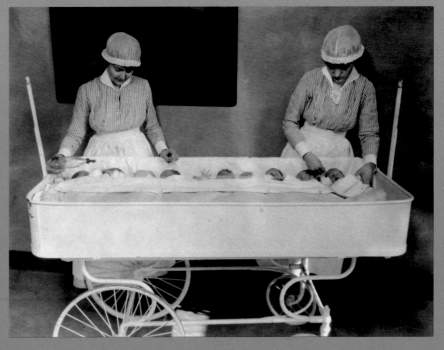

Circa 1890—*(left)* As the century turned, modern surgical practices were only beginning to arrive in the United States. In 1890 at Bellevue, an operation performed in the patient's ward room illustrates some of the progress of the day and also how far surgery had yet to go. In this procedure, ether is slowly being administered to spare the patient pain. That's progress. So is the fact that nurses, who had previously been excluded from the operating room, are seen just beginning to play their integral role. But the surgeons are still in street clothes. Their hands are not protected by rubber gloves—the gloves would not arrive for a few years yet. There are no masks. Infections from this operation were still a strong possibility.

Circa 1890—*(above top)* Exercise classes at the New York Foundling Hospital.

Circa 1920—*(above bottom)* At New York's Bellevue Hospital, several infants are packed into a single huge baby carriage, carefully tended by two nurses.

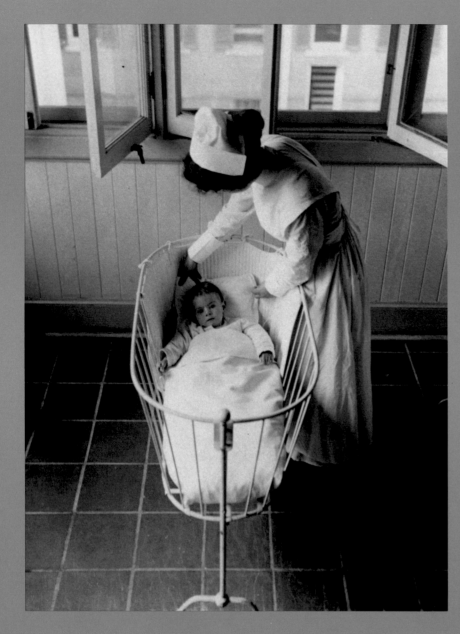

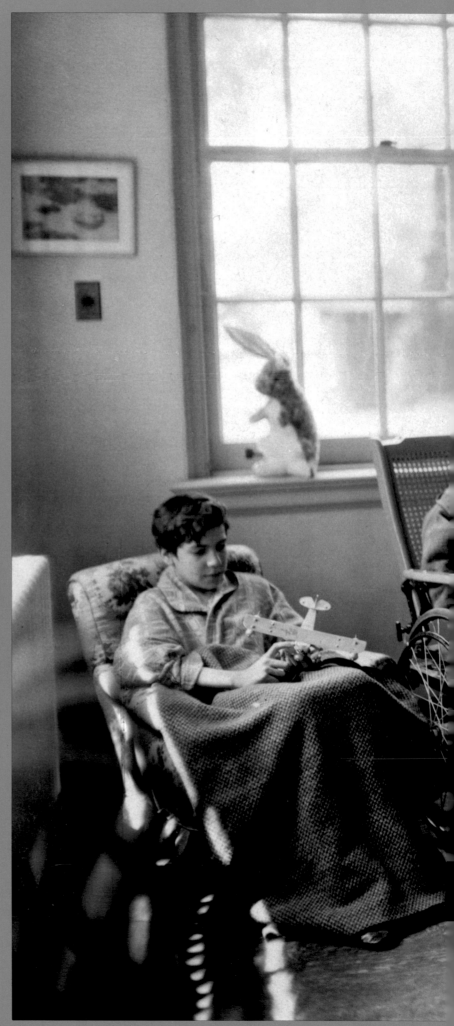

Circa 1920—*(above)* The care of children became a central part of hospital activities. Children were being born and cared for in ever greater numbers at institutions like Toronto's Hospital for Sick Children.

1932—*(right)* Young patients at Children's Hospital, Minneapolis, Minnesota. Hospitals made a special effort to create friendly surroundings for their young patients, as can be seen from the toys in this ward.

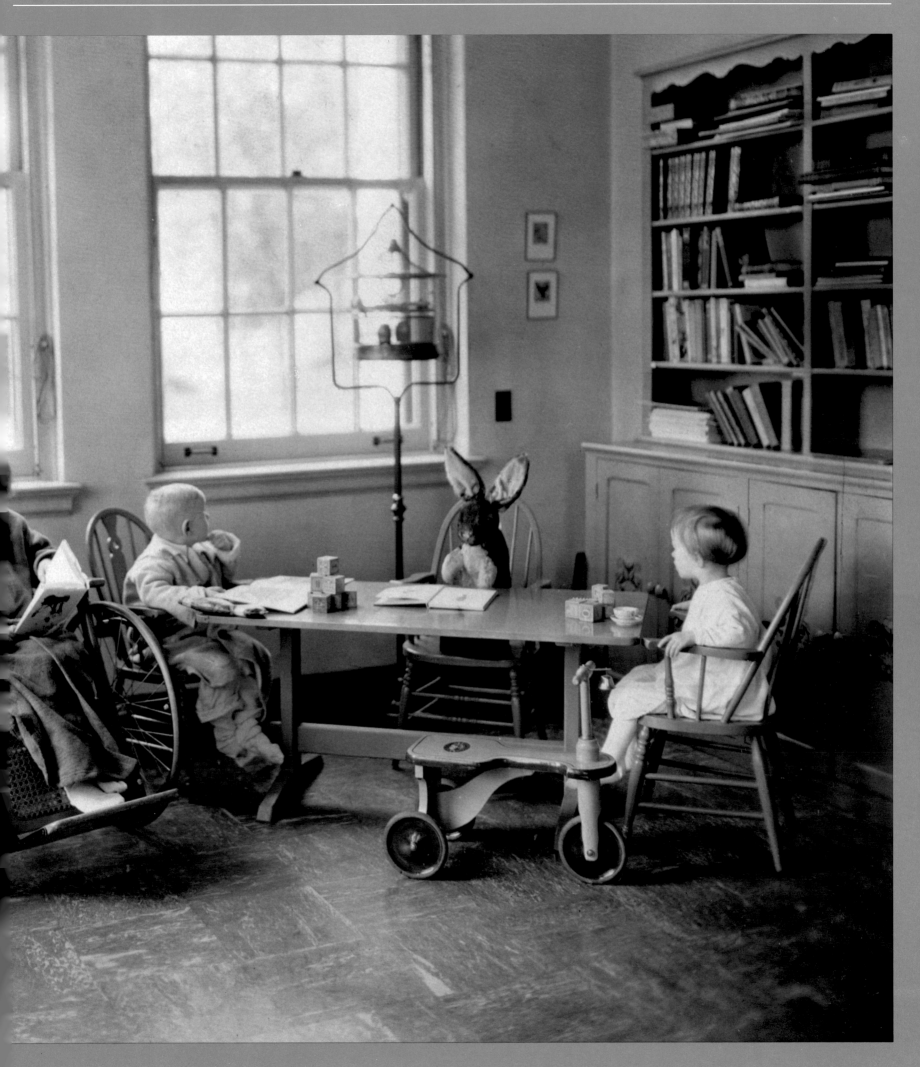

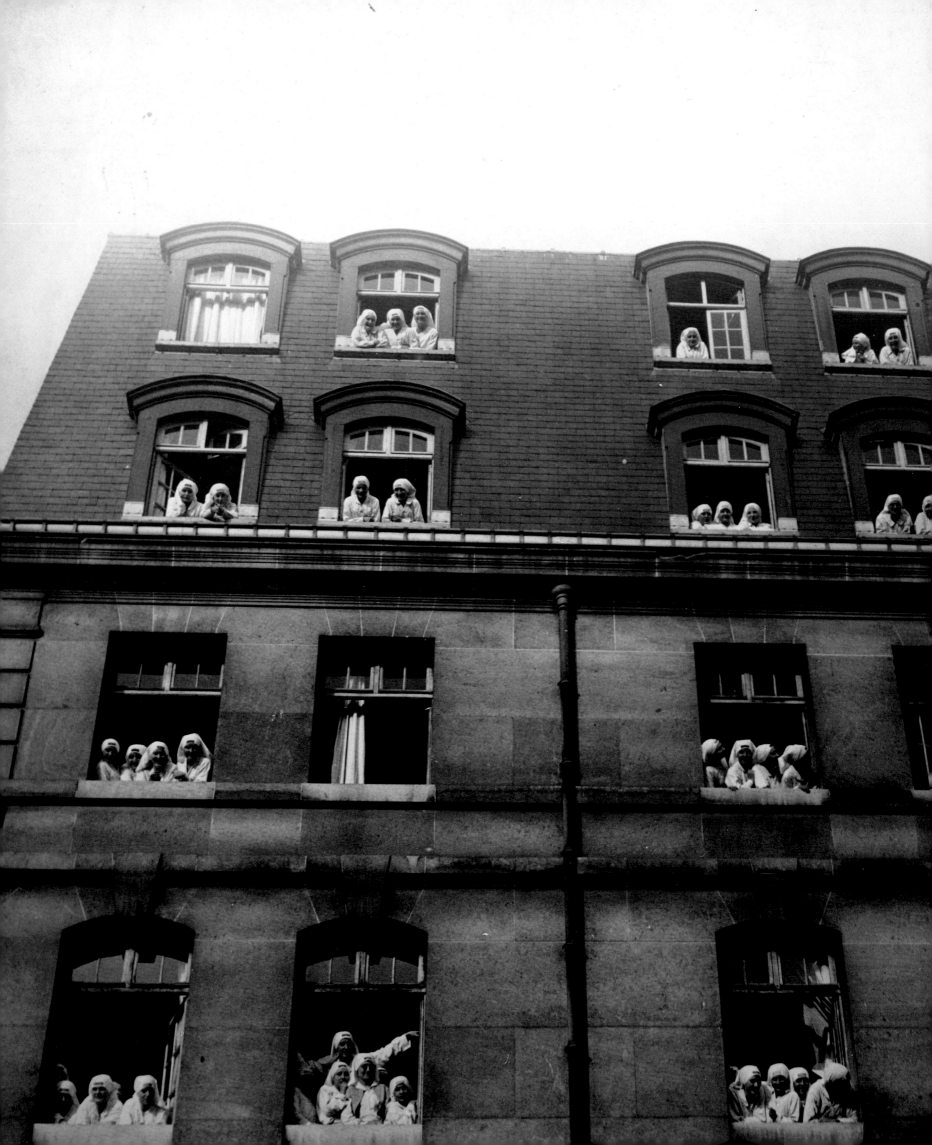

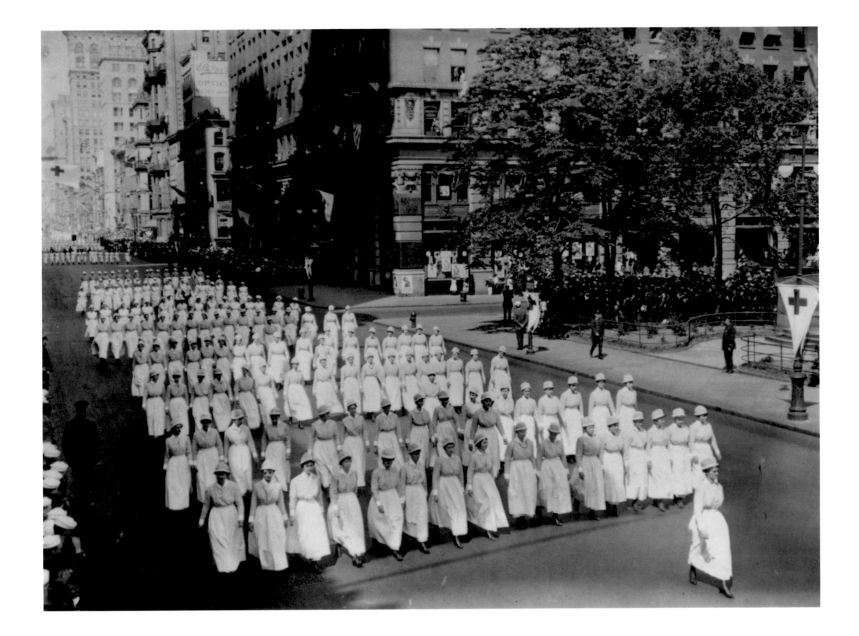

Circa 1930—*(opposite) Nurses leaning out windows, France. What is a nurse? Several hundred years before Christ, the medical philosopher Charaka already had an idea, listing four key characteristics the nurse possessed: knowledge of the manner in which drugs should be prepared, cleverness, devotion to the patient, and purity.*

1918—*(above) Graduating nurses from Bellevue Hospital School of Nursing marching on Fifth Avenue. President Woodrow Wilson observes from the right.*

1920—*(right) Nursing, as an honorable and necessary pursuit, truly took hold in America with the establishment of training schools; by 1892 there were four hundred. Here the proud issue of the New York Hospital Training School for Nurses poses in the institution's courtyard.*

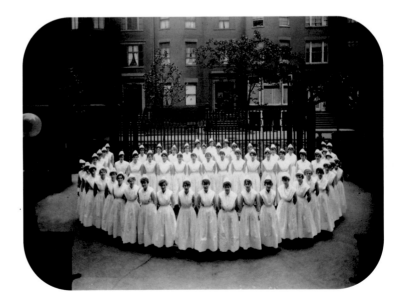

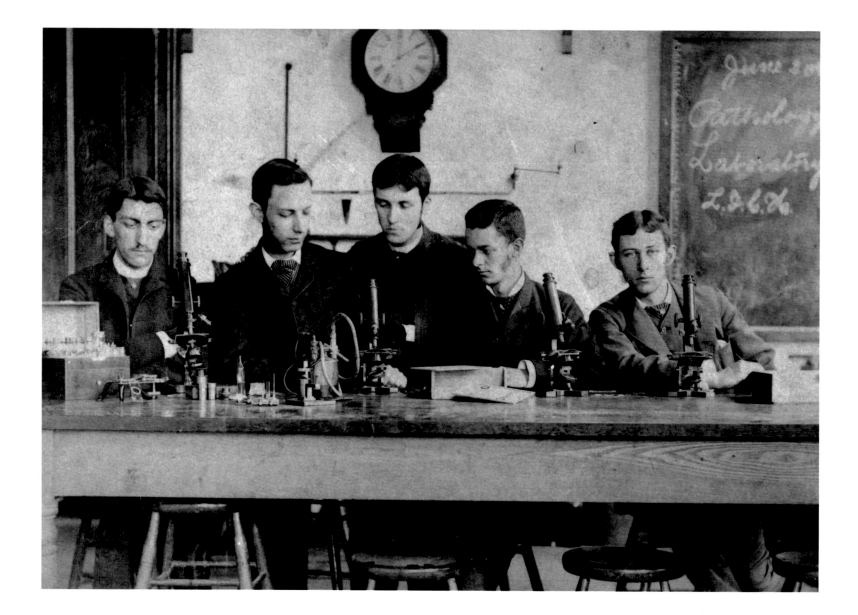

1883—(above) At the Long Island College Hospital labs, researchers joined in a stunning new pursuit: the investigation of the origin and diagnosis of disease in a laboratory. The image of the physician was changing; now he was a scientist who knew how to use a microscope.

1909—(right) Once, it was easy to become a doctor. In the early nineteenth century, America's four small medical schools offered a school year lasting about twelve weeks and courses that consisted simply of listening to lectures. Degrees were granted after one year. Few students were rejected for admission, and nearly all entering students graduated. Northwestern University in Chicago pioneered an extended curriculum—six months in 1859. Harvard followed in 1871 with a nine-month term and a three-year course that encouraged the widespread acceptance of stricter standards in medical education.

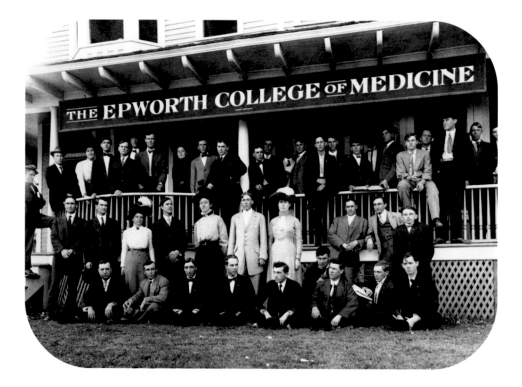

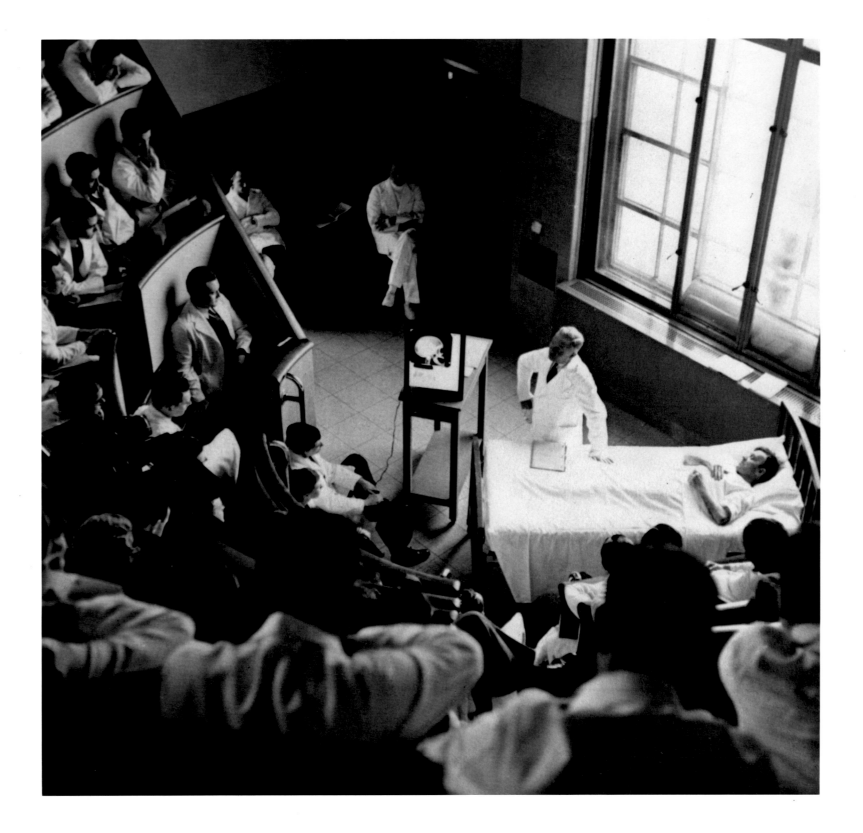

1936—*Dr. George Heuer, Surgeon-in-Chief at New York Hospital, conducts "Grand Rounds" at Cornell University Medical College, addressing the students on the subject of skull fractures.*

Circa 1888—*(following page) Before operations on live patients became a standard part of medical education, cadavers were used; here, a professor of anatomy gives a demonstration in the "bull pit" at the University of Rochester.*

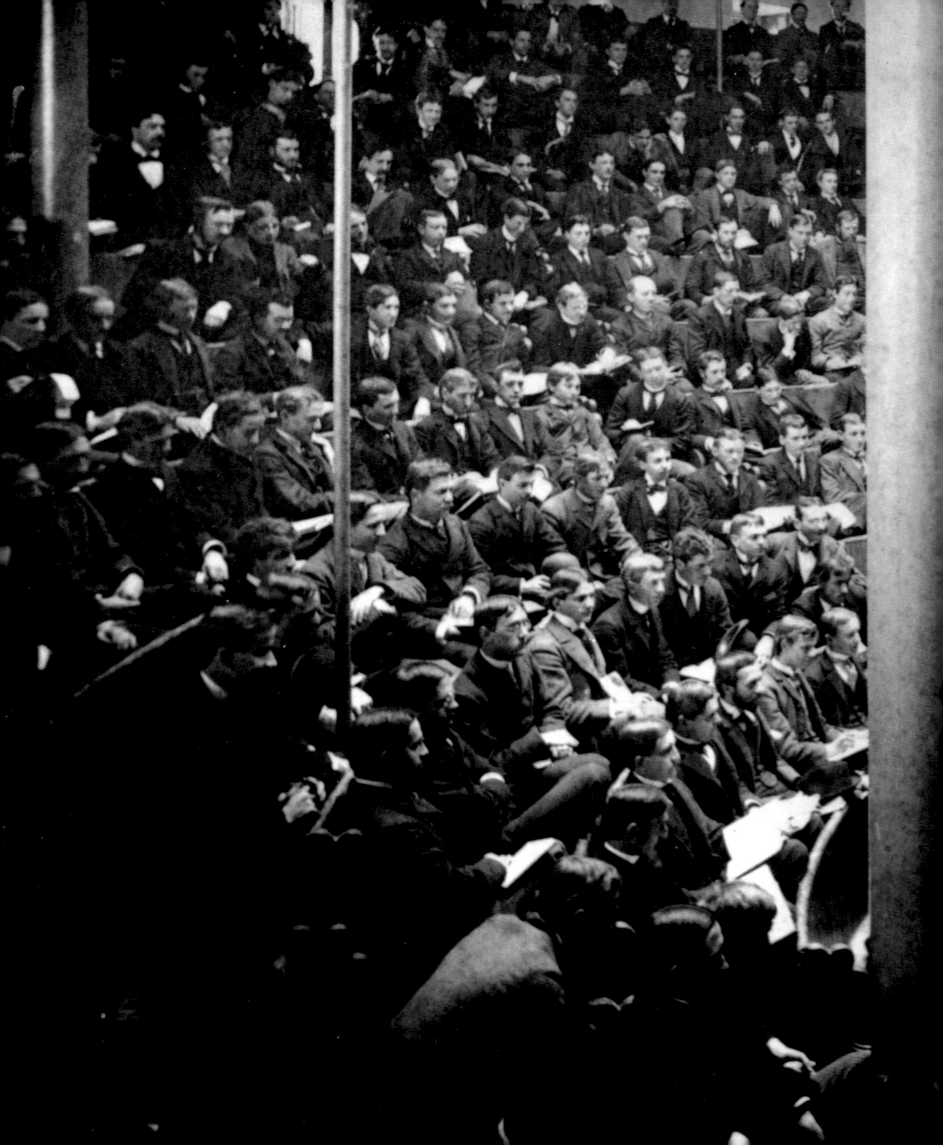

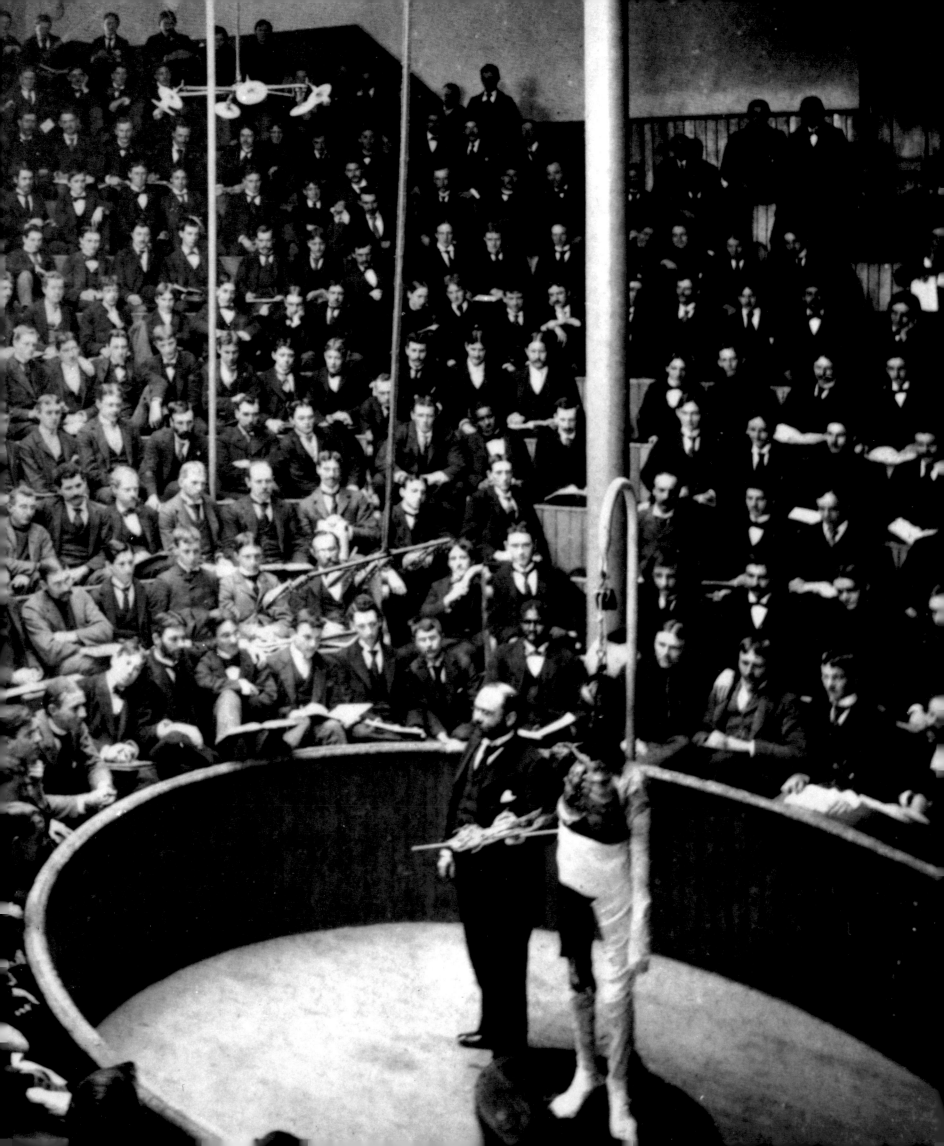

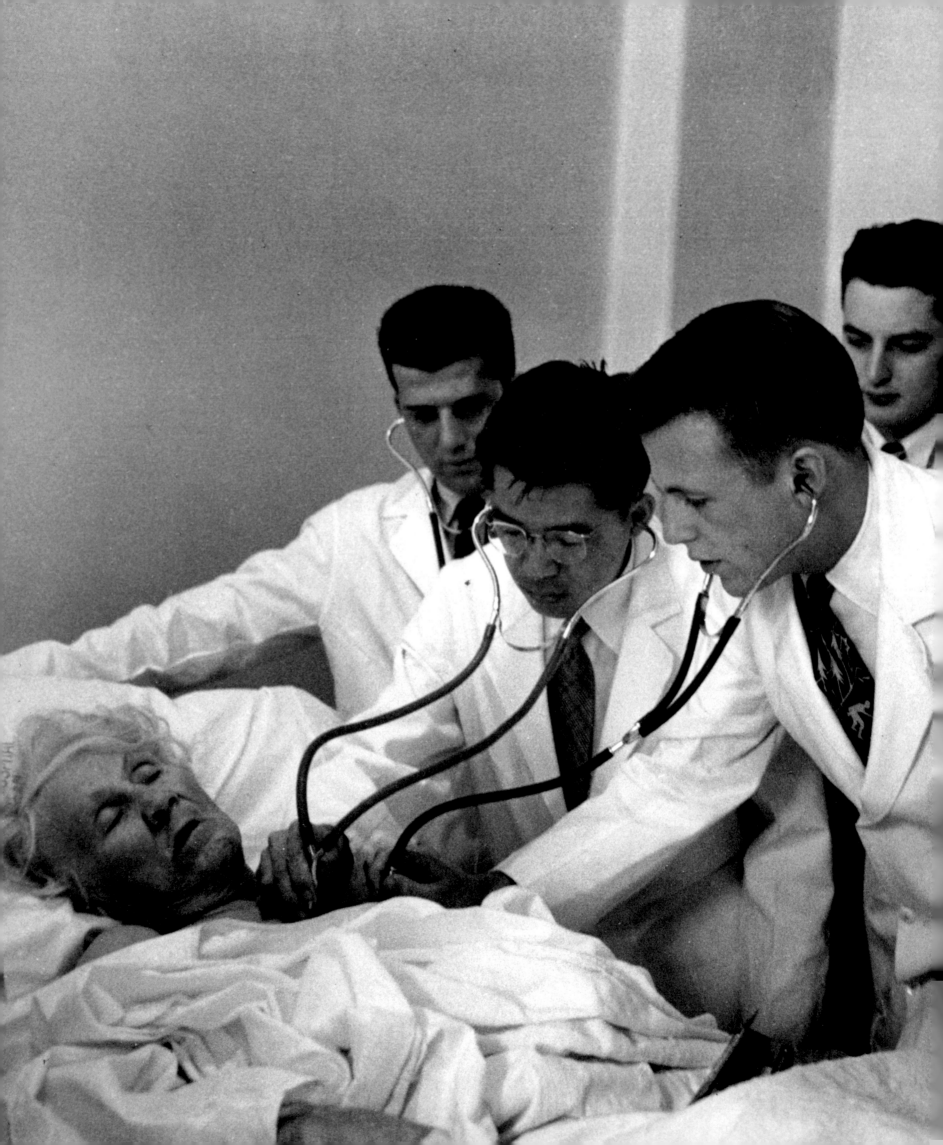

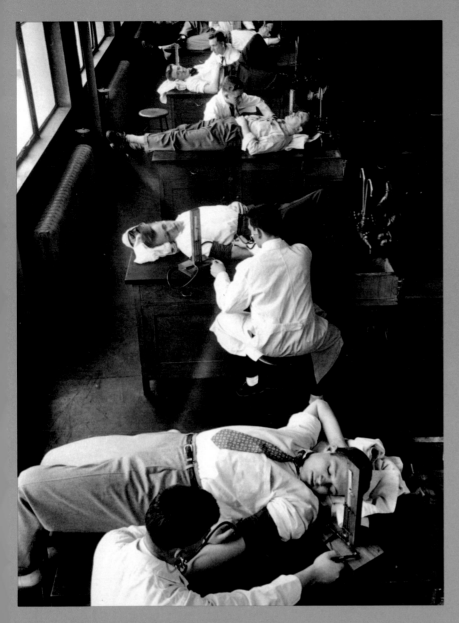

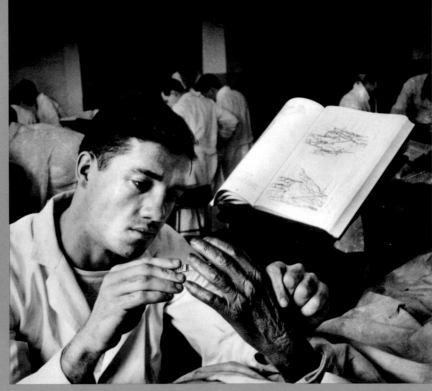

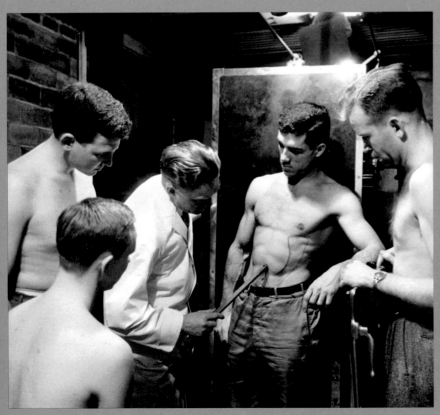

The Hard Lessons of Medical School

Nineteenth-century medical training seemed designed to keep medical students as far from the body as possible before they set off into the real world. By the middle of the twentieth century, their education was a matter of getting ever closer. Alfred Eisenstaedt, in a series of photos at the University of Michigan, portrayed the young doctors' introduction to the human body. Above, in time-honored fashion, a freshman cuts into the hand of a cadaver to trace the routes of nerves and blood vessels.

Medical schools' rising standards and strict licensing procedures stimulated American scholarship. By the mid-twentieth century, the path to becoming a physician became a grueling professional challenge. The stethoscope *(opposite),* simple and intimate, is still central to the doctor's art. Armed with that tool, sophomores at the University of Michigan's medical school get the chance to see patients, observe symptoms, and attempt a diagnosis.

Students examine their fellow students, who take the role of patients *(top left).* One of them, *(bottom left),* turns himself into a living lesson on the size and outline of the human stomach. First, the student drank barium so that his colleagues could see his stomach projected on a screen with an X-ray device called a fluoroscope. Then an anatomy professor traced the stomach's outline for the benefit of the others.

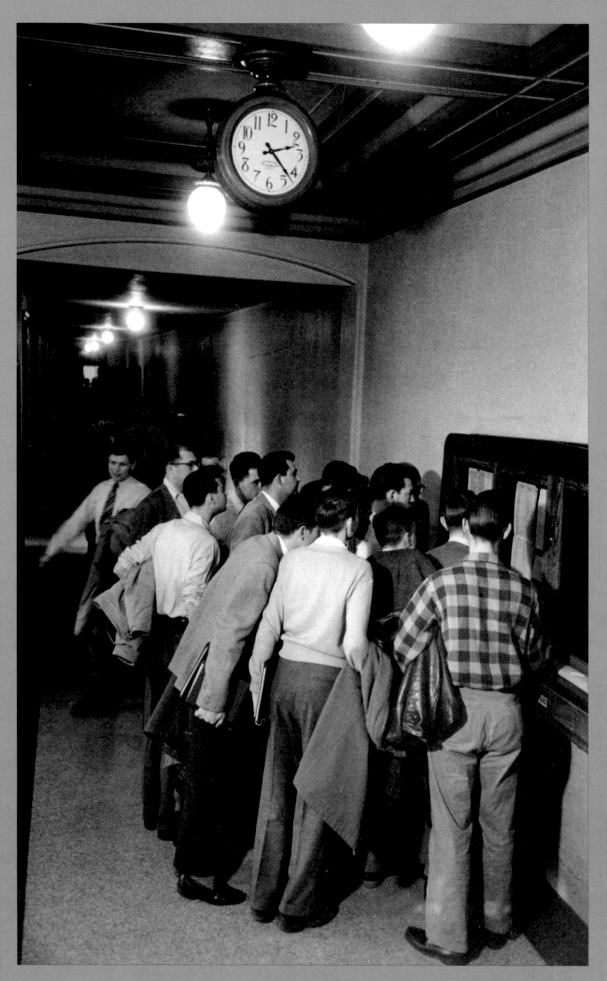

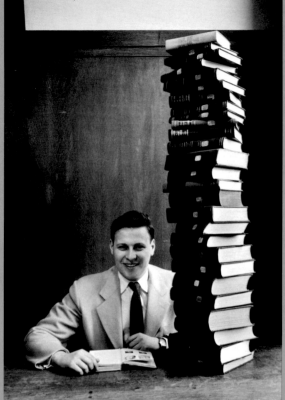

By now, medical school had taken on its modern reputation as a fiendishly difficult place to succeed. Michigan freshmen gather anxiously around the bulletin board to check their grades *(left)*. A student makes light of the heavy reading *(above)*. And in the anatomy room *(right)*, students gather for lunch, a respite from the grueling day. Work is never very far away, if only in the person of the skeleton known as Ford.

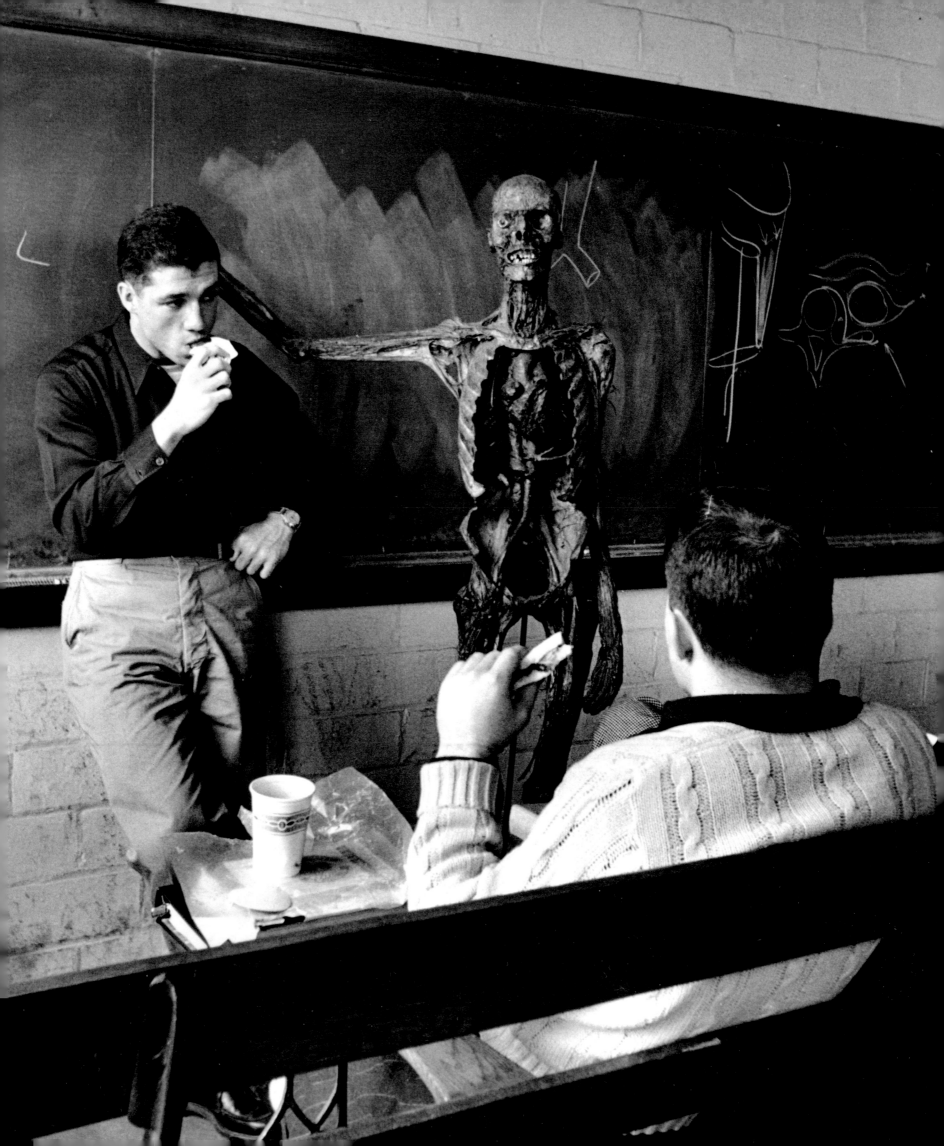

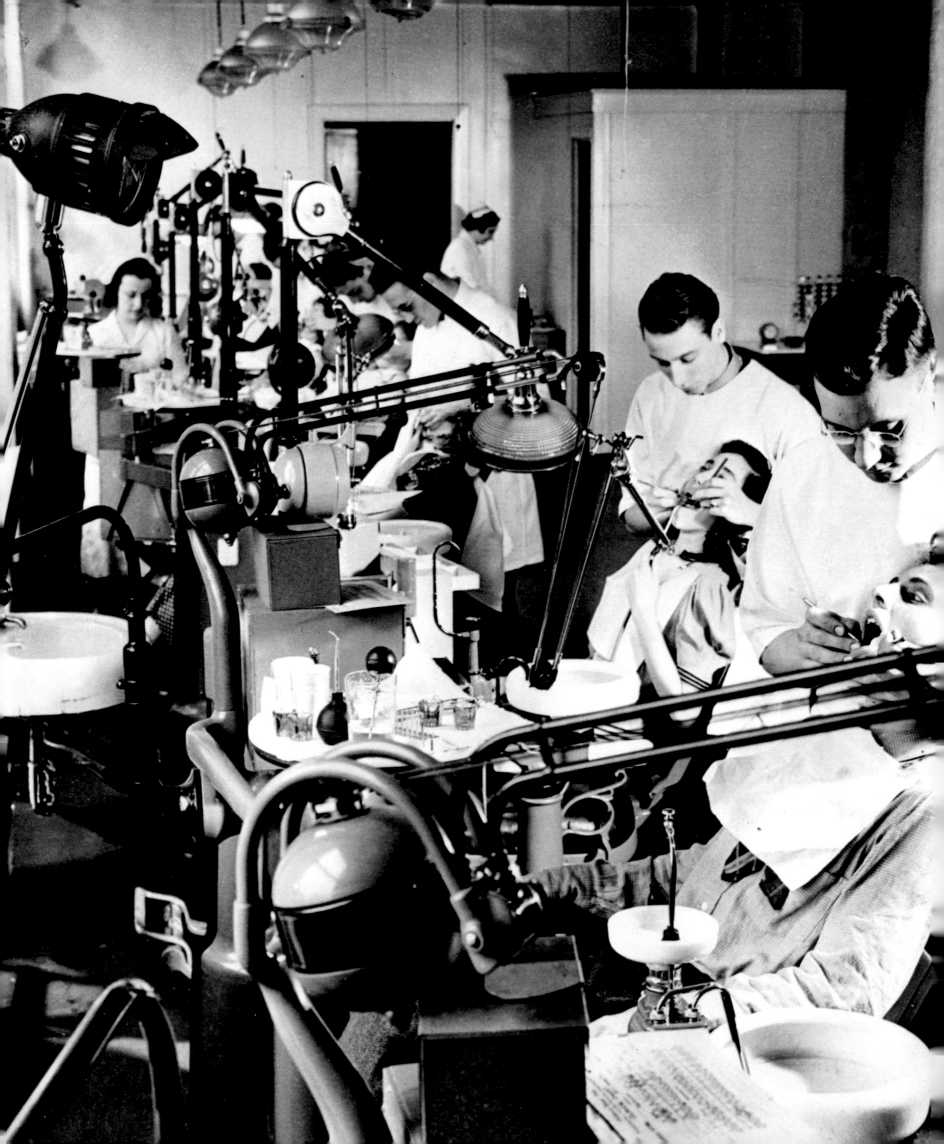

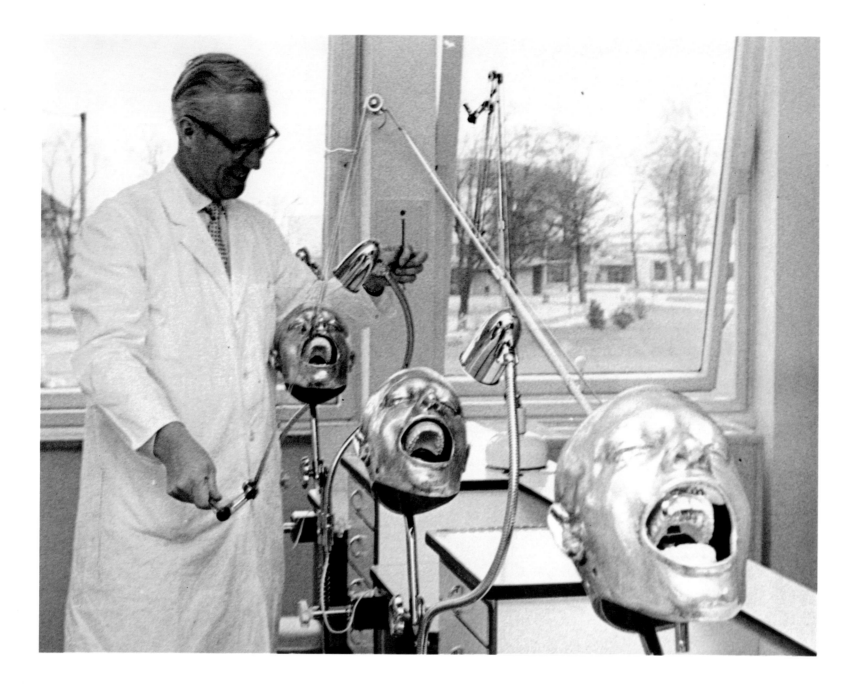

1938—(opposite) Dental clinic, Philadelphia.
Photographed by Ritake.

Circa 1960—(above) If medical students need to use
the whole body, the dentist does not: above, at the
dental hospital of the University of Bonn, "phantom
heads" used in the instruction of dental students stand
in a row, agape and ready for practice surgery.

in medical studies, he experienced some sort of conversion that has
left medical historians wondering. It might have happened in
Vienna. Somehow, at any rate, Halsted became deeply absorbed in
scientific surgery. Upon returning to the United States to work at
Bellevue Hospital in New York, Halsted concluded that this institution was no place to practice the sort of rigorously clean surgery he
had been learning. On the hospital grounds, he erected a tent, his
own personal operating pavilion. It was not cheap—it cost $10,000
in the currency of the 1880s, raised independently by Halsted and
his friends—because it required hot water and gas and a fine wooden
floor. The pavilion created quite a stir and, incidentally, drew
considerable attention to the need for aseptic conditions.

Sadly for Halsted, this was also a period in medicine that
had just discovered the miracles of cocaine. A Vienna Medical
School researcher, Karl Koller, had found that cocaine applied

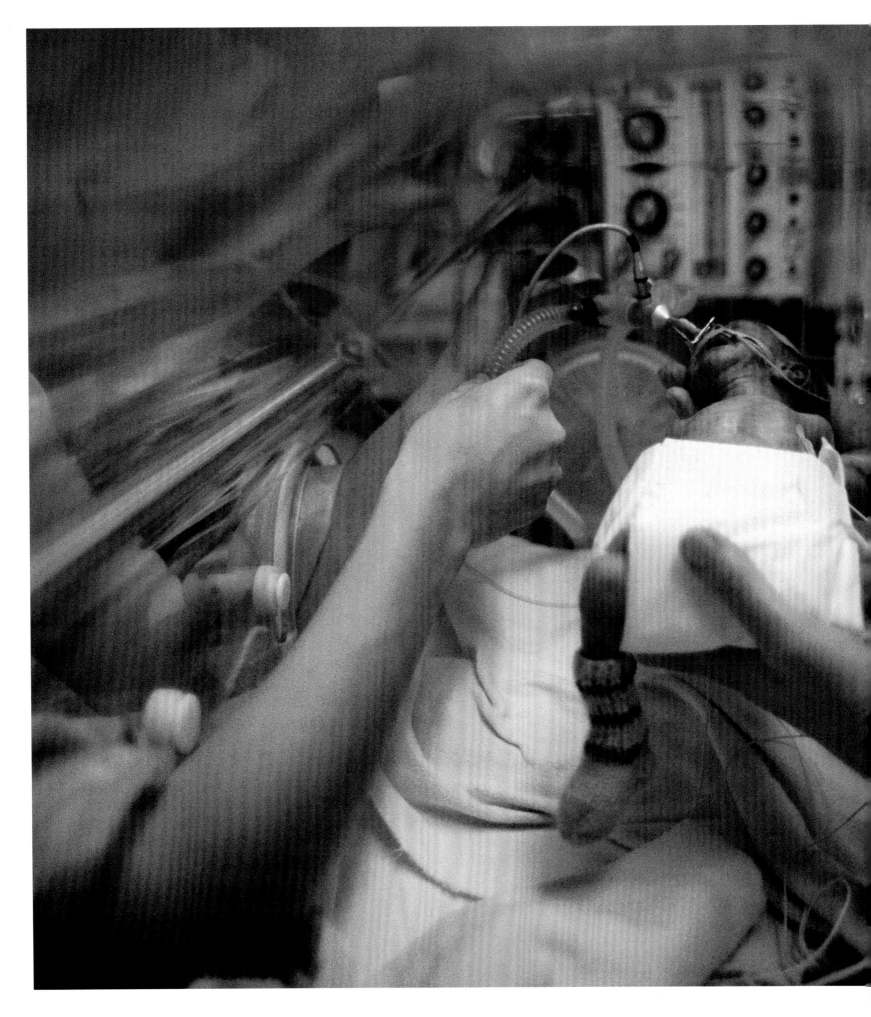

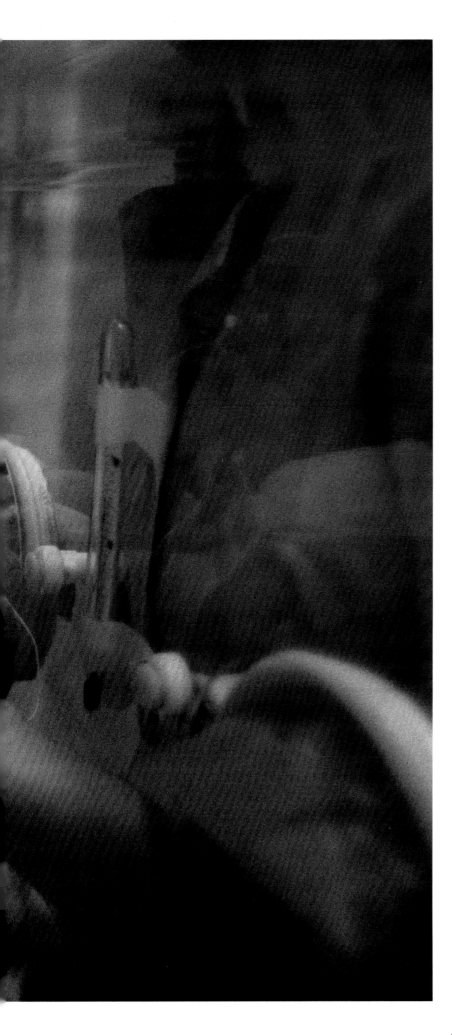

gently to the eye would allow surgeons to operate there. The young neurologist Sigmund Freud was looking into cocaine's other potential benefits (to his own eventual detriment). Halsted, along with some of his friends, stumbled on the fact that cocaine had certain recreational attributes. In time, his capacity to work declined, his mind lost some of its edge. He was addicted for the rest of his life to cocaine. Friends lied to help him out, and it was decades before the full story of his dependency emerged.

By the time the slender, balding, immaculately dressed surgeon arrived at Johns Hopkins to begin the work that would promulgate everything that he now believed, he was no longer the vigorous person he had been before with the ebullient personality, the wonderful sense of flair. Now, if you were one of his students standing by as he operated, you struggled to hear him as he mumbled. And yet he proved himself to be a magnificent teacher and managed somehow to struggle on. He taught surgeons to go easy in the body because it would heal better if they were gentler. He taught them the virtues of understanding the body so well that they could be exquisitely precise in their cutting.

Among his other achievements, Halsted studied the problem of hernias—dangerous then and often recurrent after surgery—and came up with a surgical procedure that would make that particular malady practically trivial, a procedure that would endure throughout the century. He also devised the radical mastectomy, seen as a major advance in treating breast cancer, although today it is controversial and on the wane.

THE TEMPLE OF LEARNING

Johns Hopkins Hospital in Baltimore opened in 1889. In the beginning, its designers still saw a need to cope with the evils of the atmosphere, but there was also a respect for more scientific germ theory. To curtail the movement of germs from one ward to another, the new facility had no elevators. (The germs were advised to use the stairs.) Attending opening day was Margaret Billings, the sixteen-year-old daughter of one of the institution's designers, John Shaw Billings. She remembered seeing "many of father's ideas and theories, based on his practical experience with sanitation, ventilation, lighting and other problems in war hospitals. . . . Every ward had outside windows, sunlight and fresh air, no dark rooms. Corners of walls and floors had been rounded so as not to provide cracks for bugs and dirt. It was a dream that had evolved slowly—thoroughly—completely—a dream to have everything as perfect as possible, built to last, and planned as far ahead as it was then possible

1987—*Medicine's ability to nurture premature babies has grown exponentially in recent years. Here a "preemie" infant receives emergency care, minutes after birth. Photographed by Thomas Stephan.*

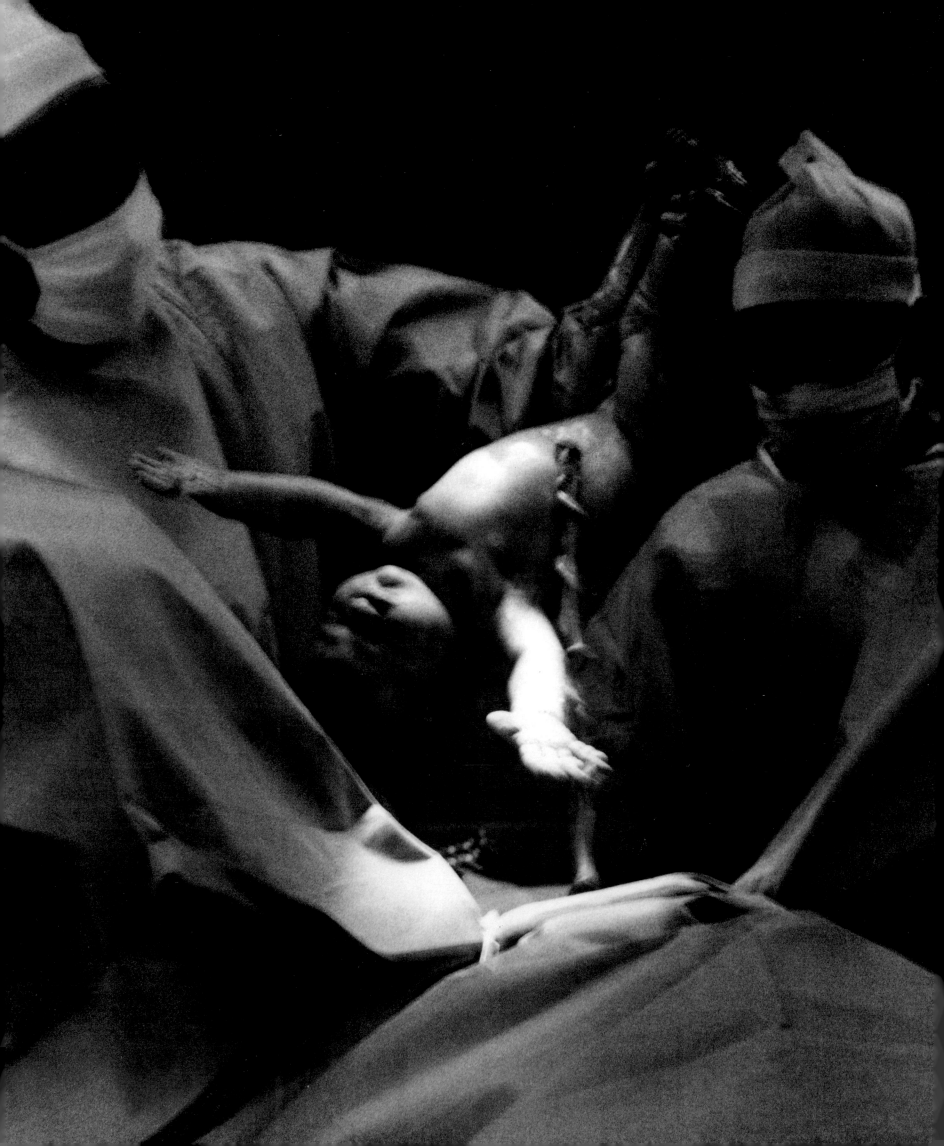

1979—*(opposite)* Birth. *Photographed by George Krause.*

1952—*(right) At the Hôpital Lariboisière, Paris, a doctor takes a moment's rest after delivering his seventh baby of the day. As childbirth moved from home to hospital during the twentieth century, it was initially only poor women, unable to afford a doctor or midwife, who gave birth in the institution. In the early decades, hospital births, which involved occasional surgical intervention, were not especially safer than home births. Nevertheless, increasing numbers of babies were being delivered in hospitals, in part because of the use of anesthesia in childbirth. Photographed by Jean-Philippe Charbonnier.*

Circa 1960—*(following page) Medical advances in treating severe burns prolonged life in a way that was unthinkable earlier in the century. Burn specialists like these in Paris became a vital part of the expanding field of emergency medicine. Photographed by Wenil Field.*

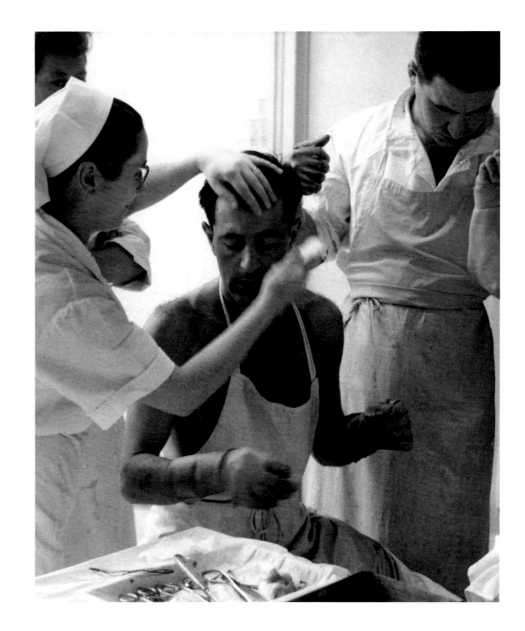

to see." It was a visionary moment in medicine.

Although sophistication in surgery and medical treatment was accelerating in Europe and at a number of sites in the United States—preeminently Philadelphia, New York, and New Orleans—Johns Hopkins was something extraordinary: a place where great forces in medicine and surgery were joining together to flow in an ever-widening stream through the twentieth century. With great apprehension, Hopkins set up stern, then-revolutionary admission requirements for its medical school candidates; a B.A. and knowledge of German and French were essential. The initial fear was that no one would apply.

If nothing else, the instructors at Johns Hopkins must have been a tremendous draw. In addition to Halsted, there was William Osler, celebrated as an outgoing and dynamic teacher. He saw to it that students got close to the patients (direct experience with patients had been denied many students in the nineteenth century

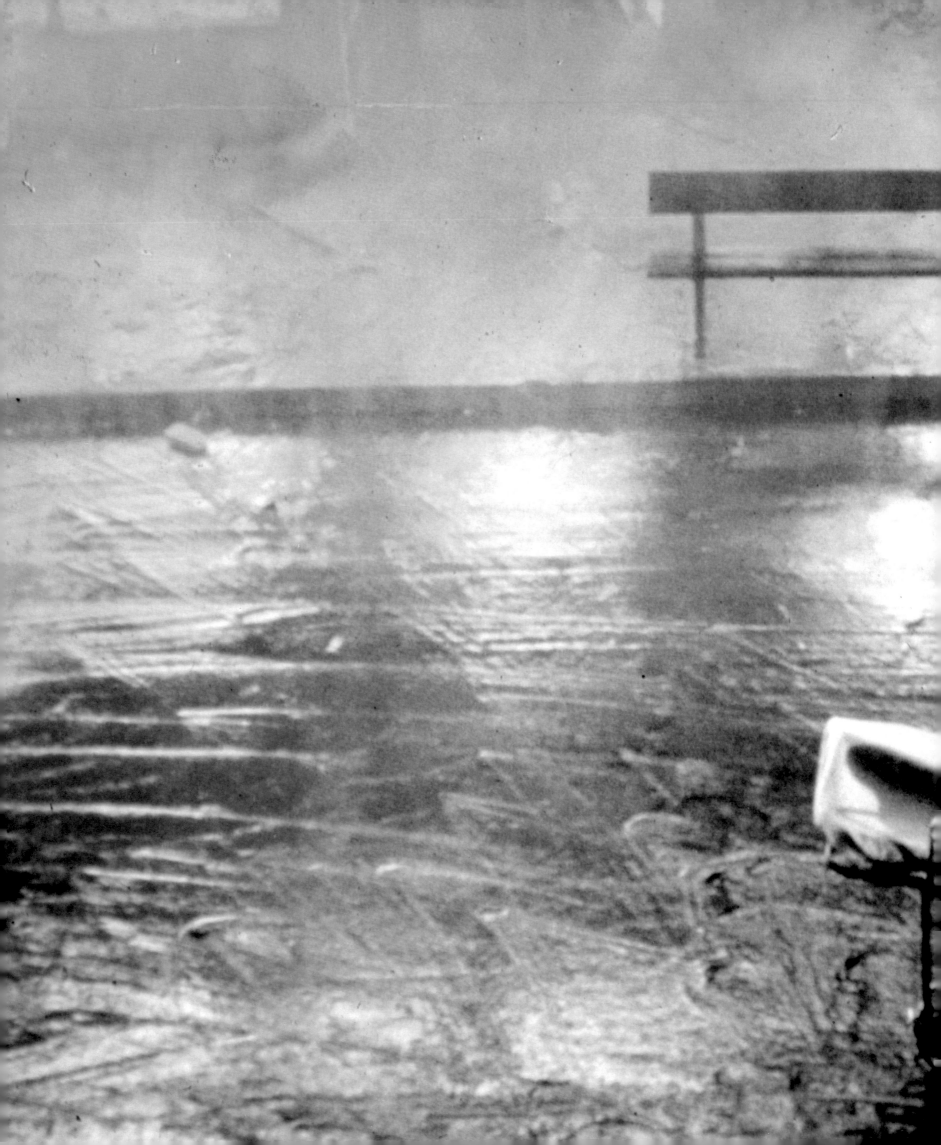

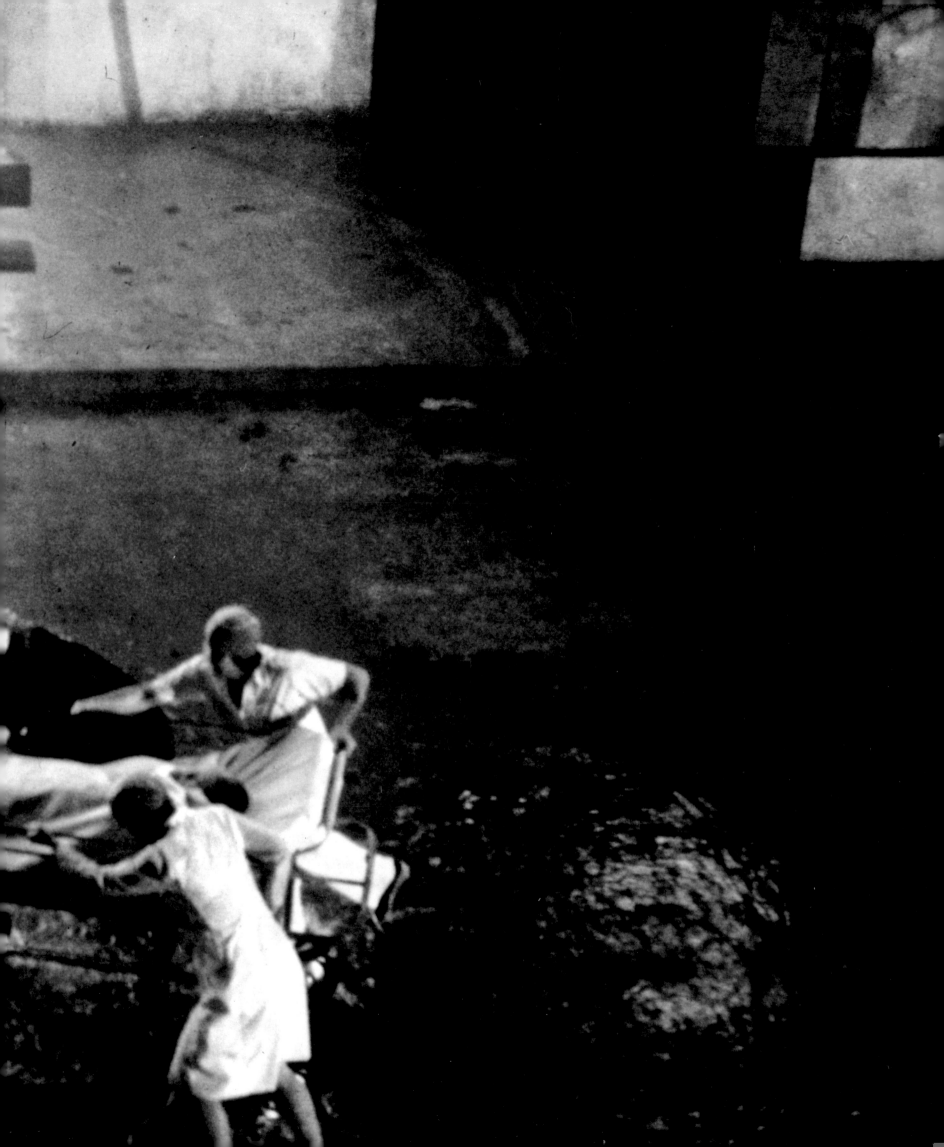

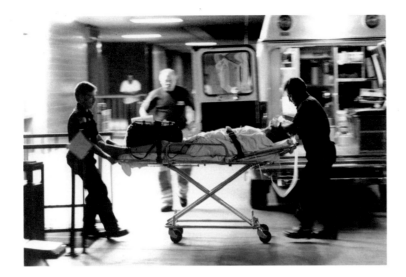

throughout Europe and the United States). Osler did not lecture much, preferring instead to move from one patient to another, trailed by his students as they examined and discussed the ailment at hand. Osler believed in the basics, particularly elevating diagnosis to an art that would dominate much of the practice of medicine throughout the early twentieth century. A meticulous man, he urged his disciples to hone habits of observation and description: "You can do nothing as a student in practice without it. . . . Carry a small notebook which will fit into your waistcoat pocket, and never ask a new patient a question without notebook and pencil in hand."

By the time of Halsted's death, surgery was feared far less than it had been. Using principles of an absolutely bloodless operating area, anatomically perfect dissection of each part, rigid rules about sterility, and accurate closing of wounds with fine silk stitches of every layer of tissue, Halsted's perfect technique represented then, and for long after, the acme of a surgeon's art. His success rate due to these innovations made medical history. But even early in the century there were already complaints that surgery had become too easy and was being abused, particularly with a rash of appendectomies. Today, kidney transplants and noninvasive procedures such as lithotripsy, which shatters kidney stones through the use of shock or ultrasonic sound waves, are considered unremarkable, new livers are exchanged for old, and hearts and lungs are outfitted with plastic replacement parts. Meanwhile, surgeons have become so adept at their craft that some procedures are done out of

---

1990—(above) *Pomona Valley Hospital emergency department. Paramedics and firemen rush into the emergency room with a patient in respiratory distress. Photographed by Elsburgh Clarke.*

1986—(right) *Charity Hospital, New Orleans. The emergency room at the changing of the shifts: understaffed, overburdened, and sometimes overwhelmed, the modern emergency room sits at the center of a maelstrom of sickness and injury in the cities. Photographed by Andy Levin.*

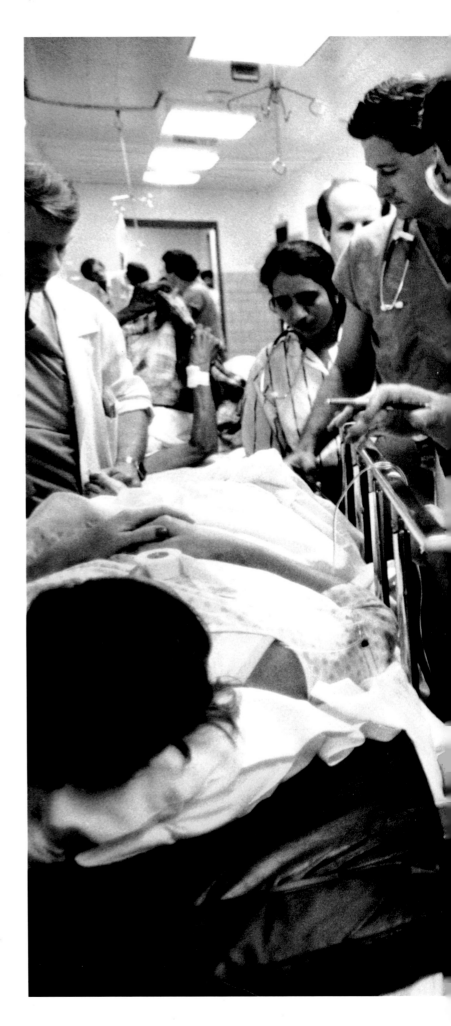

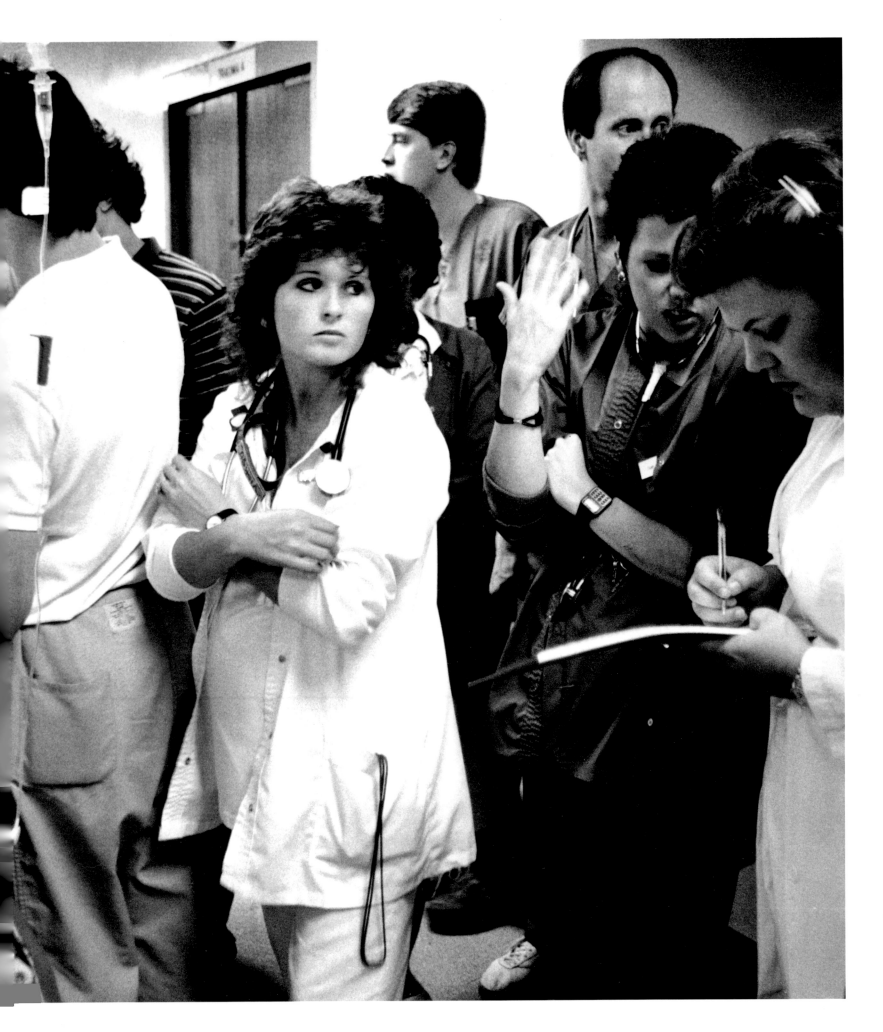

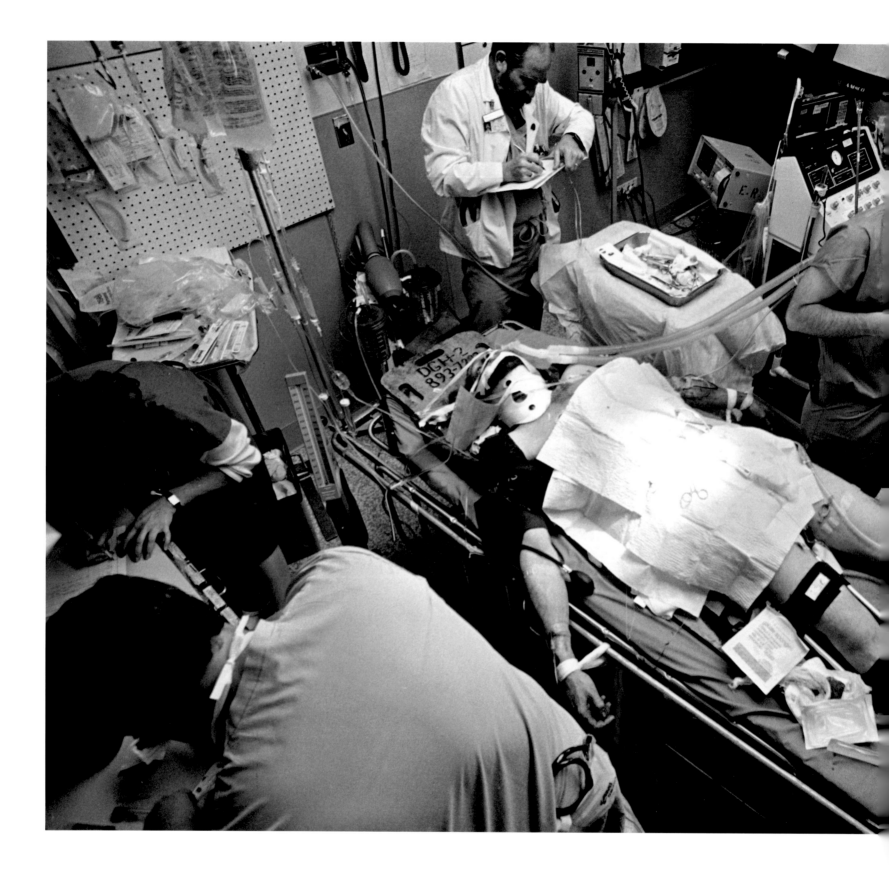

1989—*(above and opposite) Emergency room, Denver General Hospital, Denver, Colorado. "Paramedicine and EMS is different from anything else in medicine. Our attitude is different. When we have to be aggressive, that's the way we are. At times it's unorthodox, very impolite. At times we don't take people's feelings into consideration. The problem is when you're dealing with life and death, you don't have time for that. The reality is that about twenty percent of our society cannot or will not care for themselves, so the rest of society have got to make a decision about whether or not they are going to pick up the tab for that twenty percent. A lot of our patients do not have resources or have insufficient resources and we're the end of the line for them. So we have to decide what kind of society we want to live in." Paramedic quoted in* The Knife and Gun Club *(1989, Atlantic Monthly Press). Photographed by Eugene Richards.*

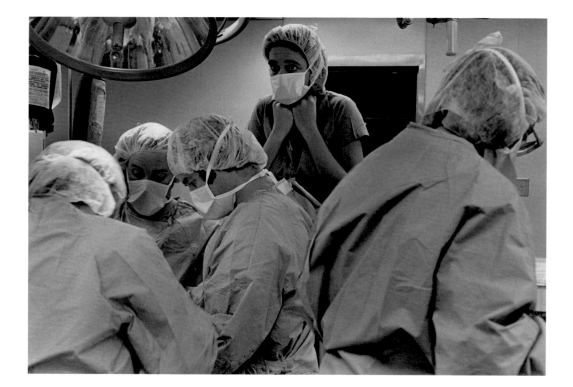

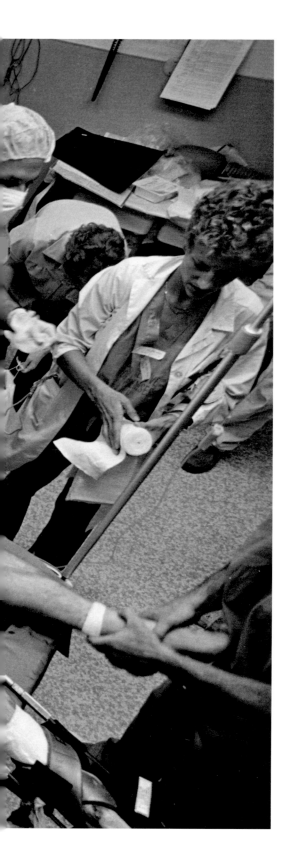

choice instead of necessity. Well-remunerated surgeons are even asked to operate simply to help the patient look better, by performing nose jobs, facelifts, and scores of other procedures intended to correct perceived failings of nature. Imagine the response a hundred years ago if you had suggested major surgery, cutting into the body, for cosmetic reasons.

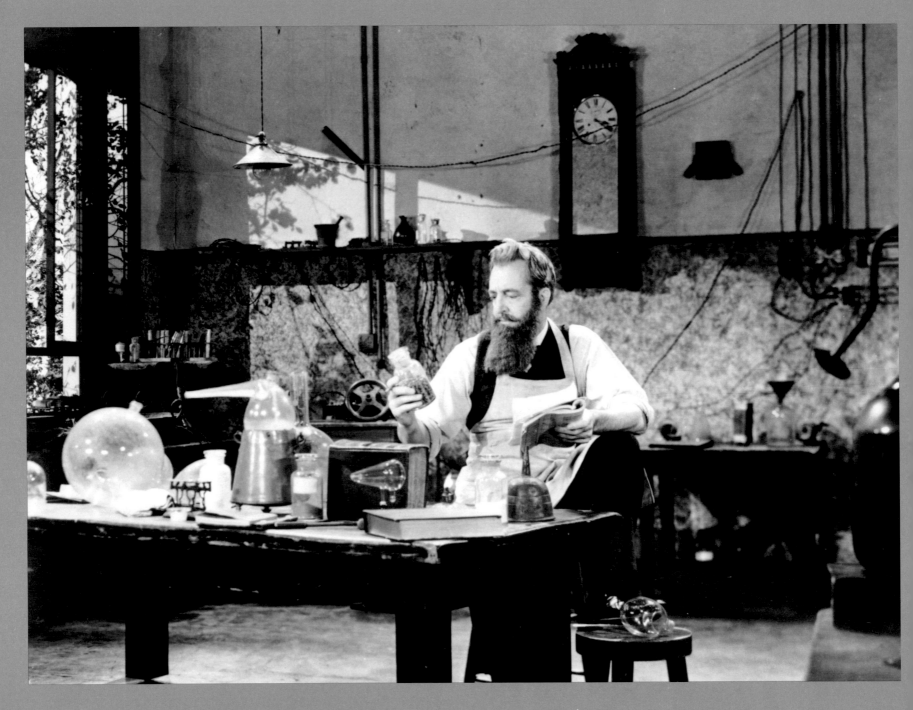

Medicine's Heroes

It is less fashionable now than it once was to single out individual medical researchers for heroism in the field. Many disputes through the years over who really deserves credit for a particular breakthrough have led to a heightened sense of caution and professional modesty. Also, medical research today generally requires so much money and so many researchers to achieve important findings that lionizing one researcher over another can leave an incorrect impression. But a glance back over the past does reveal solitary medical heroes—or perhaps pairs of them—who left a mark on medicine so bold that it is indelible, so remarkable that their names are forever tied to the advances they achieved.

Wilhelm Konrad Roentgen (1845–1922), then professor of physics at the University of Würzburg, discovered the X ray in 1895, and his findings were immediately embraced for diagnostic purposes. The X ray soon became a staple in most of the progressive hospitals worldwide by the early twentieth century. Interestingly, Roentgen's discovery launched much new construction of medical machines that later included ultrasound, pacemakers, tomography, dialysis and more. In turn, the new science of biomedical engineering was born. Roentgen, seen in his laboratory above, received the Nobel prize for his landmark contribution.

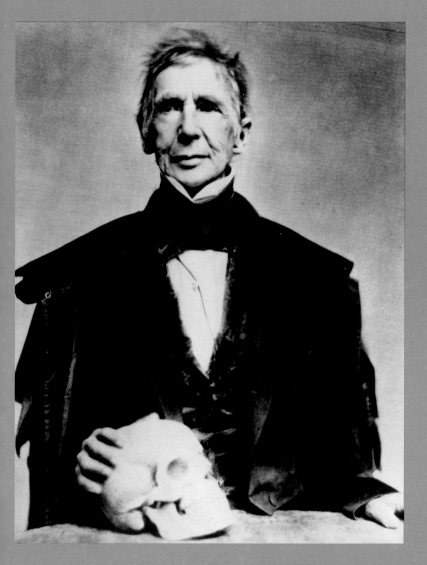

Dr. John C. Warren (1778–1856). New England today is a beacon of medical education and care in the United States and the world. But that wasn't so when Dr. Warren was teaching at Harvard in the early nineteenth-century. Warren was a puritanical, driven man who in 1799 set off for three years of medical study in London, Edinburgh, and Paris. Returning to Boston as perhaps the best-trained surgeon in the young nation, he saw a city that possessed only an almshouse to care for the sick. Warren and James Jackson, also a Harvard professor, began a vigorous and successful campaign to establish a genuine hospital for the city. In 1821 they founded the Massachusetts General Hospital, which established an association with Harvard. The hospital is today one of the world's great medical institutions, providing care for nearly two hundred thousand people a year. At his death, Warren's will called for his bones to be carefully preserved, whitened, and placed in the medical college nearby, "affording, I hope, a lesson useful at the same time to morality and science."

Dr. Harvey Cushing (1869–1939), surgeon-in-chief at Yale University Hospital, also held posts at Harvard and Johns Hopkins. He is seen standing to the left of Yale professor Otfrid Foerster. Cushing is regarded as one of the most remarkable surgeons America has ever produced. Cushing's disease, a neurological disorder whose symptoms include obesity, hypertension, hirsutism, and easy bruisability, was first described by him. Cushing was also an acclaimed author: his life of William Osler won the 1926 Pulitzer Prize in biography. But perhaps none of his achievements was more important than the promulgation of his belief that surgery must be learned on living subjects. Only then could the central concepts—diagnosis, sterile technique, careful treatment of tissues, and proper control of bleeding—be fully appreciated. Photographed by Willard Boyd.

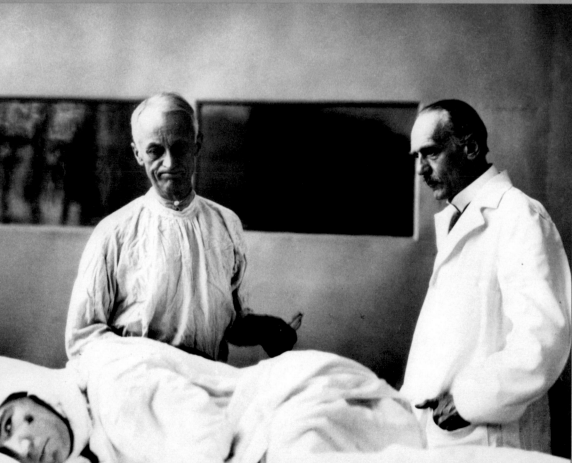

Marie Curie (1867–1934) **and Paul Curie** (1859–1906). The story of Marie Sklodowska Curie reads like fiction. Her daughter, Eve, described her mother's life vividly: "She was a woman, she belonged to an oppressed nation, she was poor, she was beautiful. A powerful vocation summoned her from her motherland, Poland, to study in Paris, where she lived through years of solitude and poverty. There she met a man whose genius was akin to hers. She married him; their happiness was unique. By the most desperate efforts they discovered the most magic element, radium.... This discovery not only gave birth to a new science and a new philosophy; it provided mankind with a means of treating a dread disease."

Although she worked in the laboratory of her husband, Pierre, Marie Curie began her work on radioactivity independently and was only later joined by her spouse. They worked alone, supported by their own funds. Marie Curie's theory that radioactivity was a property of the atom was borne out by the research. The Curies won a Nobel Prize in

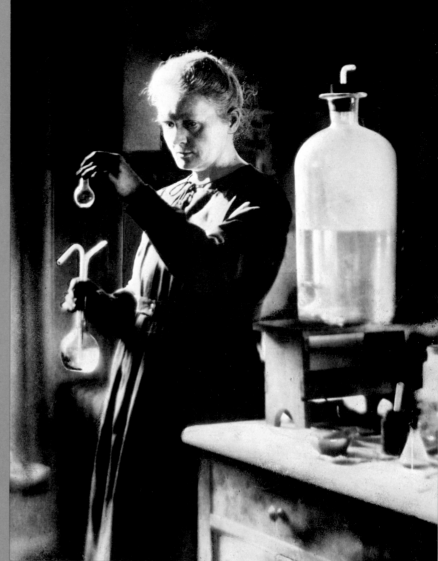

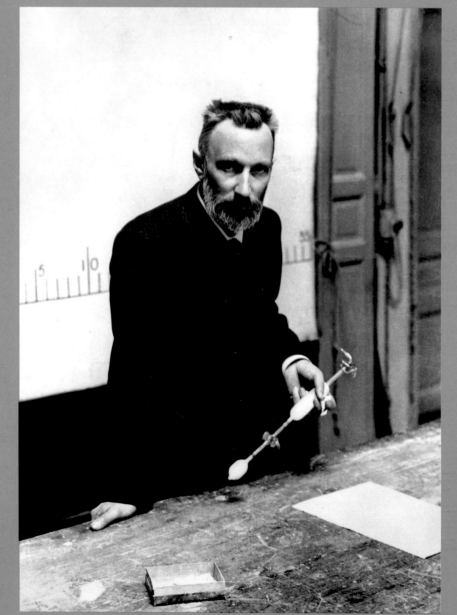

1903, along with A. H. Becquerel who discovered radioactivity itself. By 1906, radium's usefulness in treating cancers was known. The world-renowned partnership was destroyed when Pierre Curie was killed in a traffic accident while crossing the rue Dauphine. In 1911, Marie Curie won her second Nobel Prize. Today, her story endures as an inspiration for women in science.

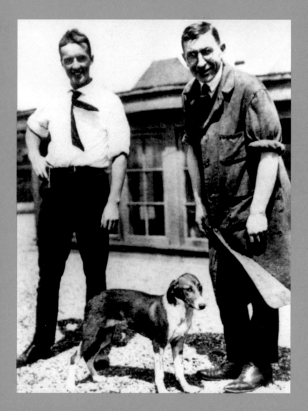

F.G. Banting (1891–1941) and **C.H. Best** (1899–1978). Diabetes could not be controlled until insulin was found. It was Frederick Grant Banting and Charles Herbert Best—working under the direction of J. J. R. Macleod—who in 1921 isolated a hormone from the pancreas that would later be called insulin. When Eli Lilly introduced insulin as a drug in 1923, a productive life finally became possible for victims of diabetes throughout the world. Banting and Best are shown here on the roof of the medical building at the University of Toronto with one of the first diabetic dogs to have been saved by insulin. Banting was killed in a plane crash in 1941 while on a medical war mission. That same year, Best became director of the Banting and Best Department of Medical Research at the University of Toronto.

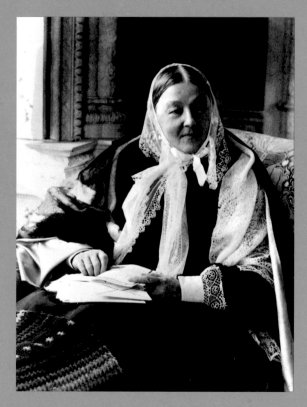

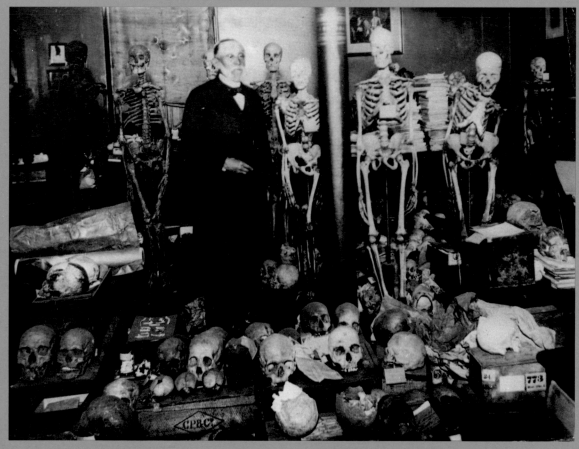

Florence Nightingale (1820–1910). By sheer force of character, Nightingale, born in Florence, Italy, created the movement that led to professional status for nurses. Her career began when she nursed her mother through a terminal illness, but her formal exposure to medicine was a three-month course at the Institute for Protestant Deaconesses in Kaiserwerth, Germany. When she took a contingent of nurses to the Crimean War, she found miles of dirty beds, no facilities or equipment to care for or feed soldiers, and a mortality rate of forty percent. Her presence alone seems to have been salutary. The soldiers responded to her with great warmth: "We kissed her shadow as it fell and lay our heads on the pillow again content." Her administrative genius and reforms saved thousands of lives. After the war, she established the Nightingale School and Home for training nurses at St. Thomas's Hospital in London. In a personal way, she paid dearly for her dedication: she contracted typhoid in the Crimea and suffered thereafter from chronic illnesses. Her tenets are basic and still profound: "The art is that of nursing the sick— please mark, not nursing sickness." Photographed here at an old-age home by Millborne of Aylesbury.

Rudolf Virchow (1821–1902). This photograph of Virchow and friends in the pathology laboratory at the Charity Hospital, Berlin, has always been used to project an image of the physician dedicated to his work. But Virchow was a man of even greater distinction than the photo suggests. A professor at the University of Würzburg and a director of the Pathological Institute, Berlin, he powerfully influenced nearly every branch of medicine. Virchow was an inspirational reformer as well, initiating a landmark, and widely imitated, sanitation movement in Berlin.

CHAPTER THREE

SPREADING THE KNOWLEDGE

CRITICS OF MODERN MEDICINE BITTERLY DECRY THE LOSS OF THE PERSONAL TOUCH AMONG TODAY'S DOCTORS. YET DESPITE THE CRITICISM THERE ARE MANY DOCTORS WHO ADMINISTER TO THEIR PATIENTS WITH SENSITIVITY AND WARMTH. SOME EVEN MAKE A GREAT SACRIFICE BY LEAVING HOME AND TAKING THEIR SKILLS TO REMOTE LOCATIONS. THESE DOCTORS WILL ALWAYS HEAR THE CALL FOR HELP.

Contemporary medicine has had to confront two prevailing popular notions about the healing arts: first, that many doctors are preoccupied with money, and second, that it is difficult, sometimes even impossible, to persuade enough physicians to work in rural or inner-city locations where they are most needed.

In the early part of the century, compassion was one of the most important parts of a doctor's service. Physicians certainly could not promise effective cures. Lewis Thomas, the physician-memoirist, recalls a conversation on medicine's limitations that he had with his father, also a physician, in 1918:

"[He] intended to make clear to me, early on, the aspect of medicine that troubled him most all through his professional life; there were so many people needing help, and so little that he could do for any of them. It was necessary for him to be available, and to make all these calls at their homes, but I was not to have the idea that he could do anything much to change the course of their illnesses. It was important to my father that I understand this; it was a central feature of the profession, and a doctor should not only be prepared for it but be even more prepared to be honest with himself about it."

Thomas' father wrote prescriptions because he knew people expected him to and it reassured them, not because he had special faith in the medications' salutary ability. He was skilled at diagnosis, so his patients had the sense that the mystery of *(continued on page 94)*

———

Circa 1946—*Resourceful German dentists managed to bring their clinics to the children: the mobile lab's window is closed so the patient can be shielded from the shouts of other youngsters.*

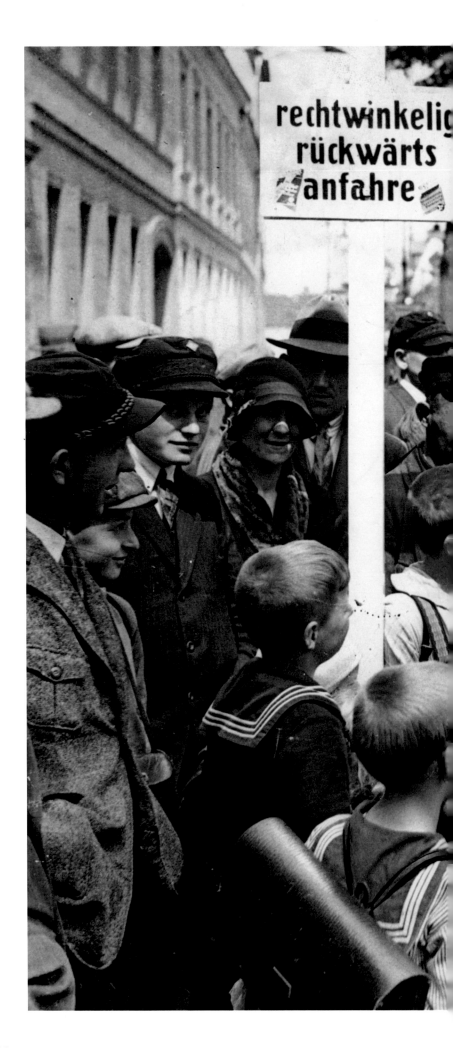

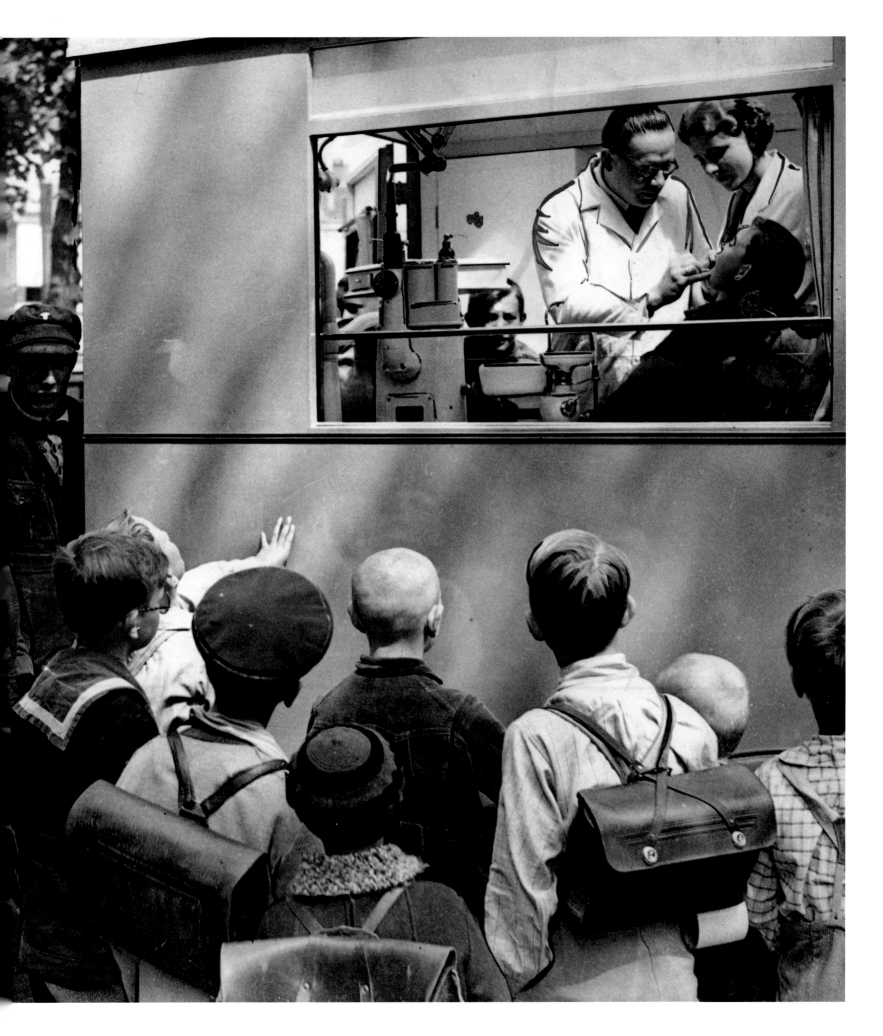

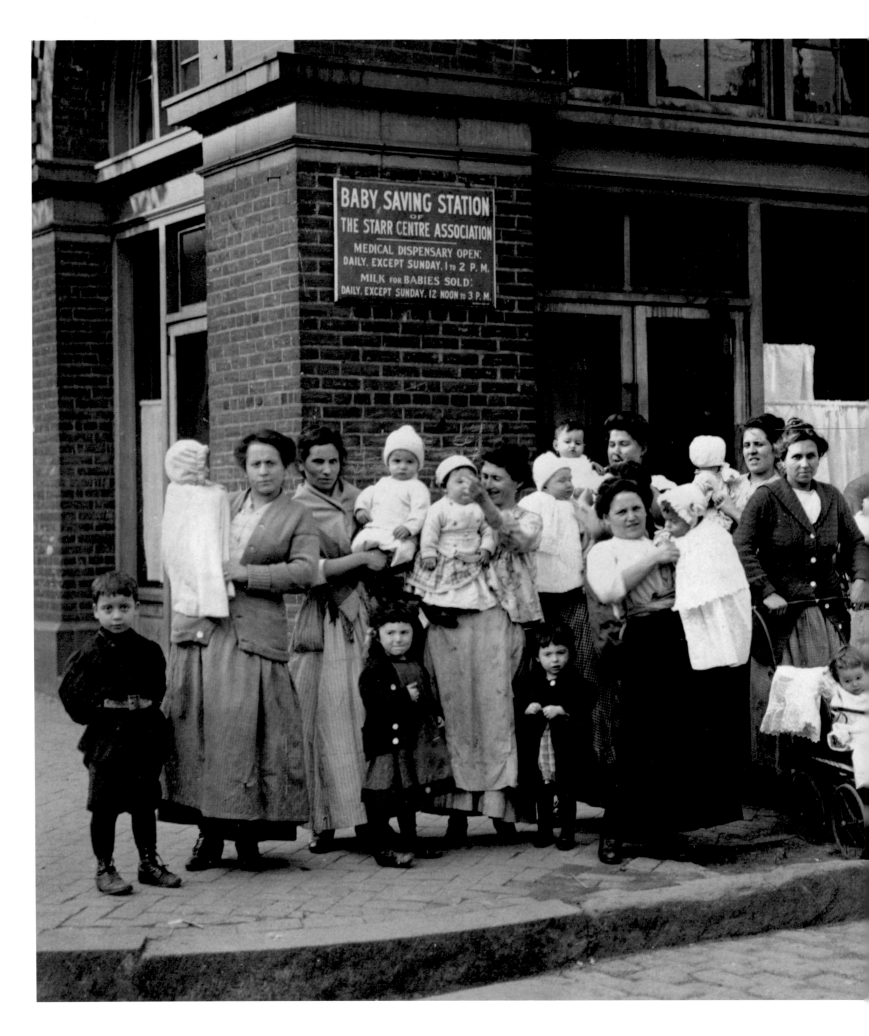

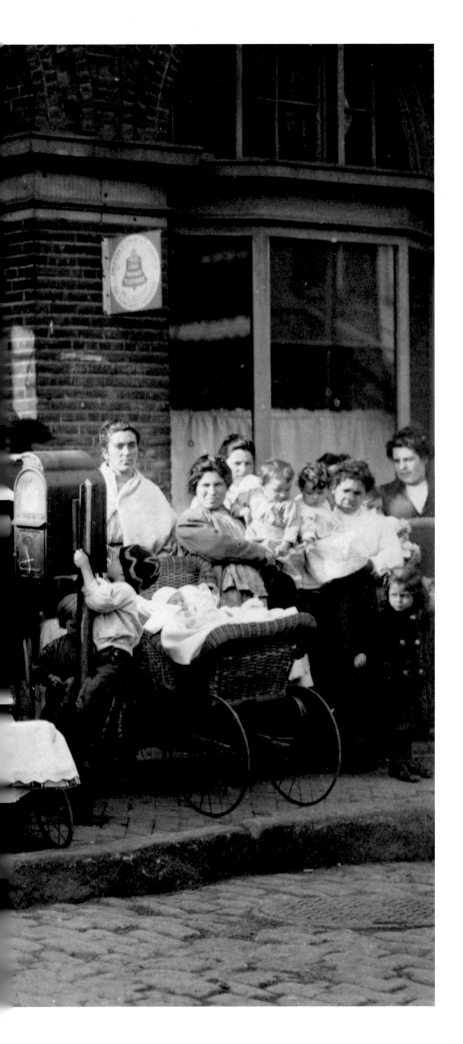

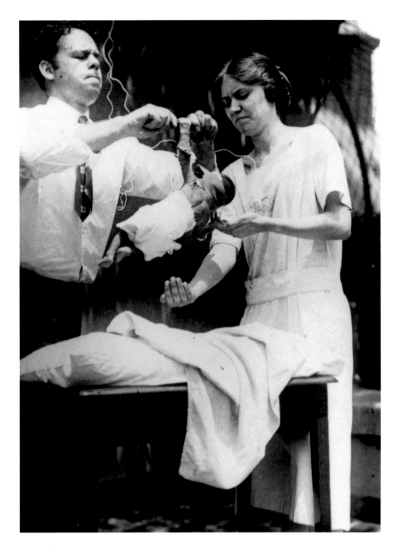

Circa 1915—*(left) An alarmingly high infant mortality rate dictated vigorous preventative efforts, including a "baby saving station" sent into slum neighborhoods of Philadelphia. Baby saving was a comprehensive program that included prenatal care, instruction for mothers in feeding and rearing their babies, sick and well baby care at local clinics, and the provision of pasteurized milk.*

Circa 1920—*(above) A Johns Hopkins physician uses a bar-grip test to investigate the reflexes of a baby supported in a sling.*

their misery was lifted, and that made them feel better.

In the decades to come, the house calls that were so much a part of the senior Dr. Thomas' practice were largely sacrificed by physicians on the altar of practicality. By 1960, house calls represented less than one percent of all doctor-patient contacts. This decline was directly tied to the migration of doctors toward group practice, hospital affiliation, and the perceived need to be nearer the technological support that doctors had come to rely on. (In today's hospitals, doctors can have a urine analysis done in seconds and read X rays on the spot.) In 1932, fewer than one percent of the active physicians in the United States felt the need to practice as part of a group. In 1975, eighteen percent did. By the nineties, so many doctors were immobile—tied to their offices and their associates— that one issue of the *Journal of the American Medical Association* contained a study and an editorial on the efficacy and advisability of helping people over the telephone. The editorial was headlined "The 'House Call' in the Electronic Era."

How one appraised these developments as they evolved throughout the industrialized West depended a great deal on personal values and personal perspective. David J. Rothman writes in *Strangers at the Bedside* that "the organization and delivery of medical care almost guarantee that at a time of crisis patients will be treated by strangers in a strange environment." He sees the new patient as a "wary consumer" rather than a "grateful supplicant." And he describes the doctor's work as now entangled in a system that brings in the government and other institutions whenever decisions are made.

Rothman observes, "In the 1930s, conversation with patients was inseparable from diagnosis and treatment, and thus it was not necessary to emphasize the need to talk to them. Three decades later such conversations were add-ons—something physicians ought to do as moral, not medical obligation."

A spokesman for the American Medical Association (AMA) asserts that medicine has reached a point where it is so complex that "no one, no matter how bright he or she is, can deal with the entire spectrum, even within their own specialty," adding, "there is a fundamental desirability in having a doctor stick to what that doctor knows best." At the same time, the AMA staunchly believes in persuading doctors to hone their sensitivity to patients.

One of the thrusts of modern medicine is a vigorous educational attempt to help today's highly specialized, highly trained, technologically competent doctors to keep people in mind. Even if they do not travel beyond the hospital or clinic, these doctors are

---

Circa 1900—*Visiting nurses, sponsored by Infant Welfare Societies, were sent directly to the homes of mothers and their children to tutor them in child care, as this nurse does in New York City. The care of children was so alarmingly poor that one in four was expected to die before the age of five.*

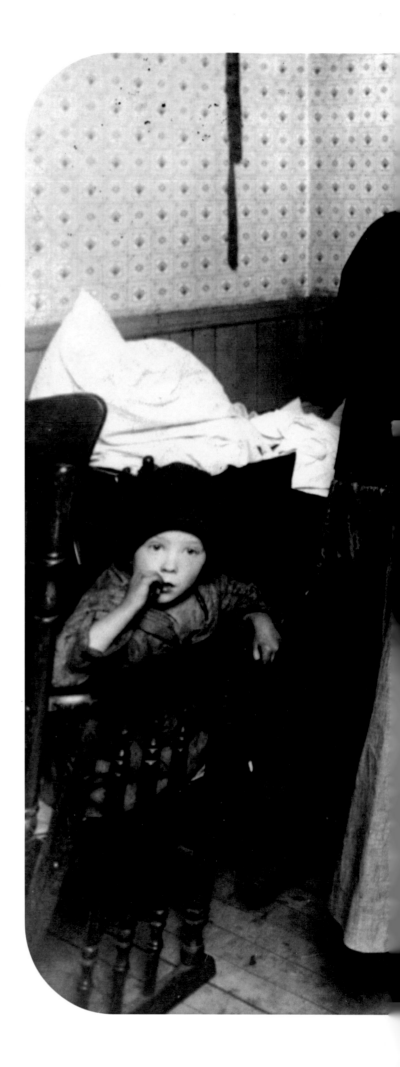

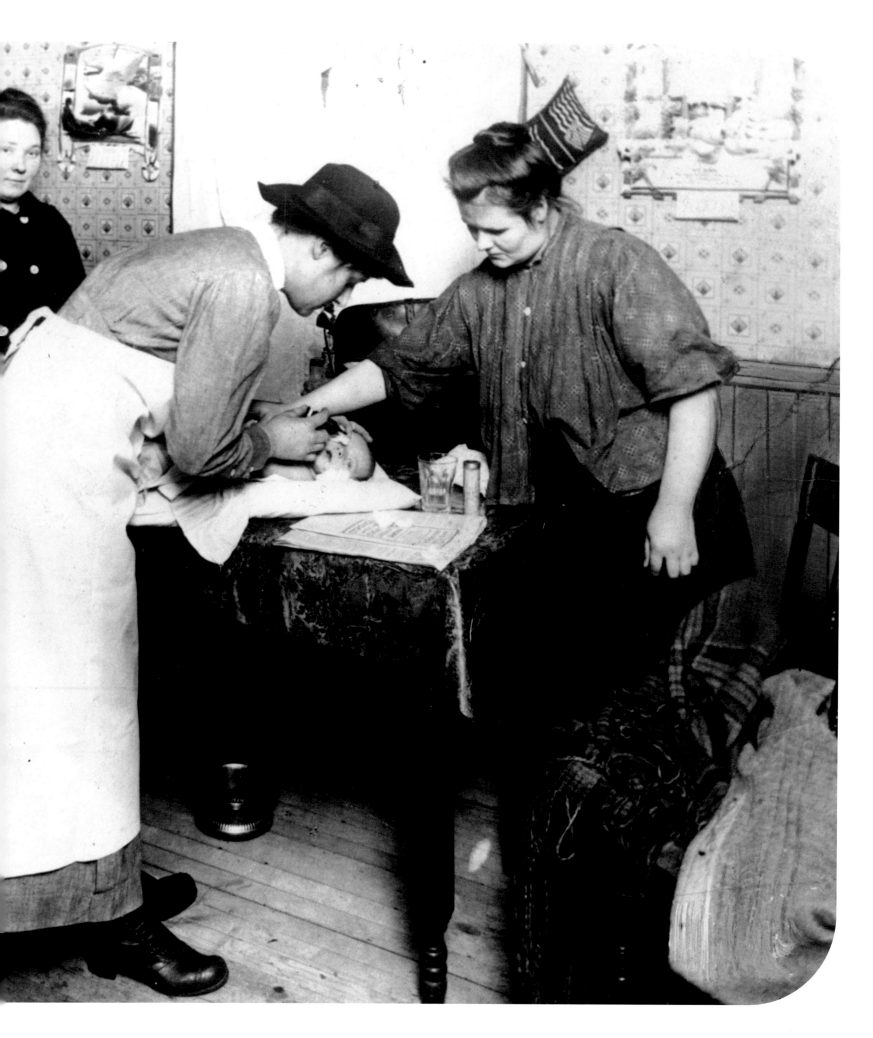

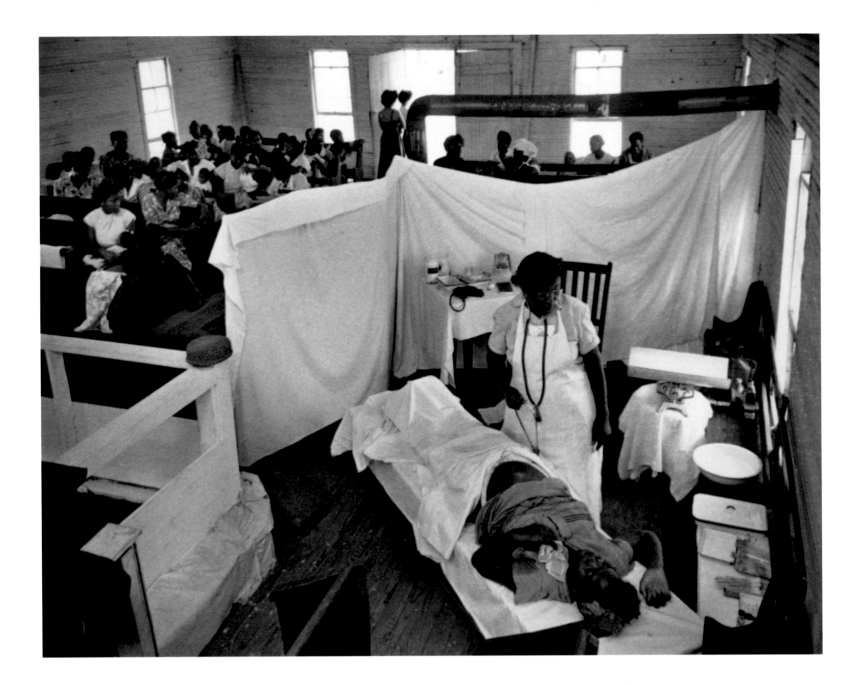

being asked to take a trip, metaphorically at least, away from the landlocked world of the technocrat and into the open ocean of compassion, into the lives of the people they must help.

At Bellevue Hospital in New York City, where the hustle, bustle, and naked horror of the urban hospital experience are evident every day, doctors are involved in a teaching program in psychosocial medicine. They discuss feelings—theirs and the patients'—and how to listen better, how to convey information better. Harvard's pioneering approach, called New Pathways, attempts to help doctors become aware of the patient's life outside the hospital and what sickness means to the rest of his or her life experience. The idea is to broaden the doctor's mind at a time when the pressures of training and then making a living are severe.

Some medical observers believed that the push toward a greater responsibility to the community would be especially influ-

1951—*(Above and opposite) Nurse midwife Maude Callen, a licensed midwife who set up a temporary clinic in an old church to tend her patients and train apprentice nurses, provided medical care and social services to over ten thousand people in a four-hundred-square-mile area in rural North Carolina. The original photo essay was published in* Life *Magazine in the issue of December 3, 1951. Public response was phenomenal, including gifts amounting to $18,500 for Maude's new clinic.*

Although at the turn of the century midwifery was common and midwives delivered most babies, by the Depression this practice was in decline. Women came to believe that medically supervised births offered advantages in safety and pain relief. In the latter part of the century, midwifery made a comeback.
Photographed by W. E. Smith.

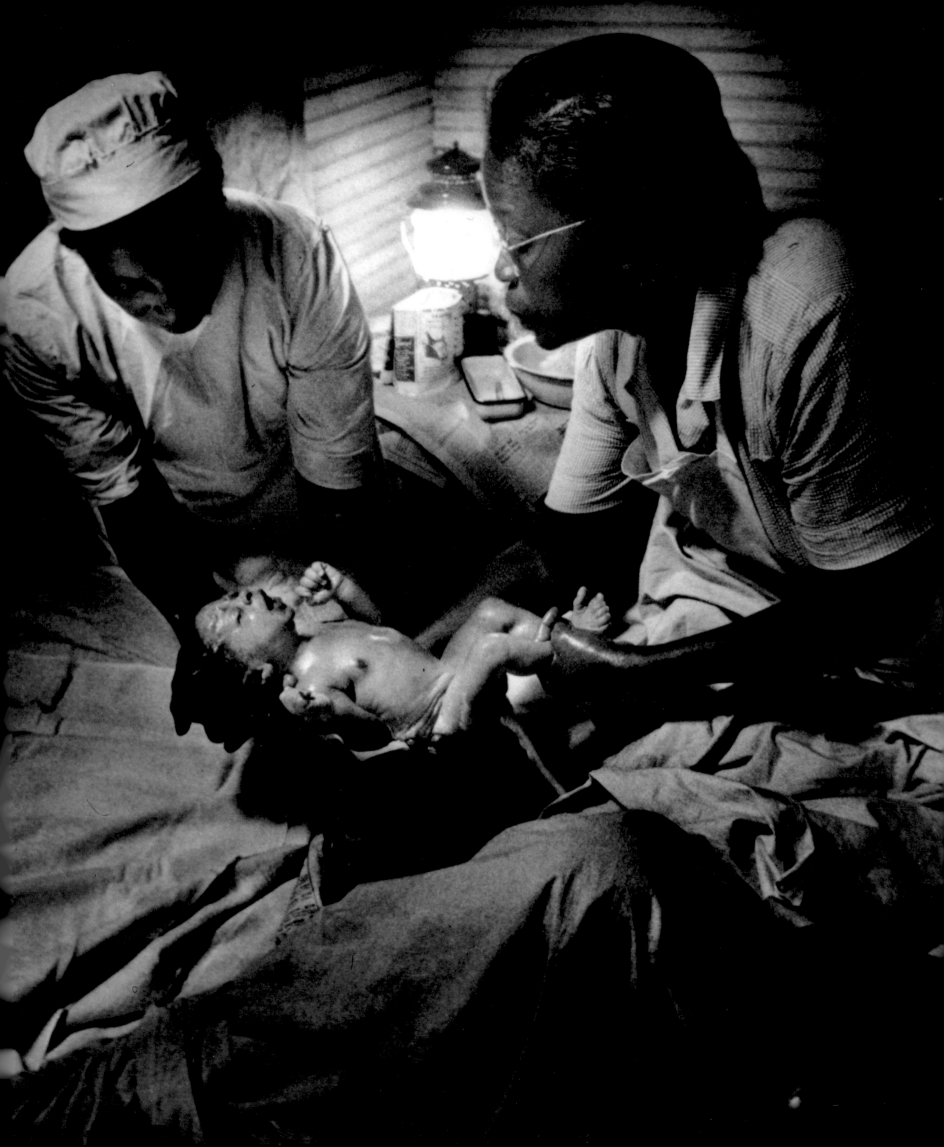

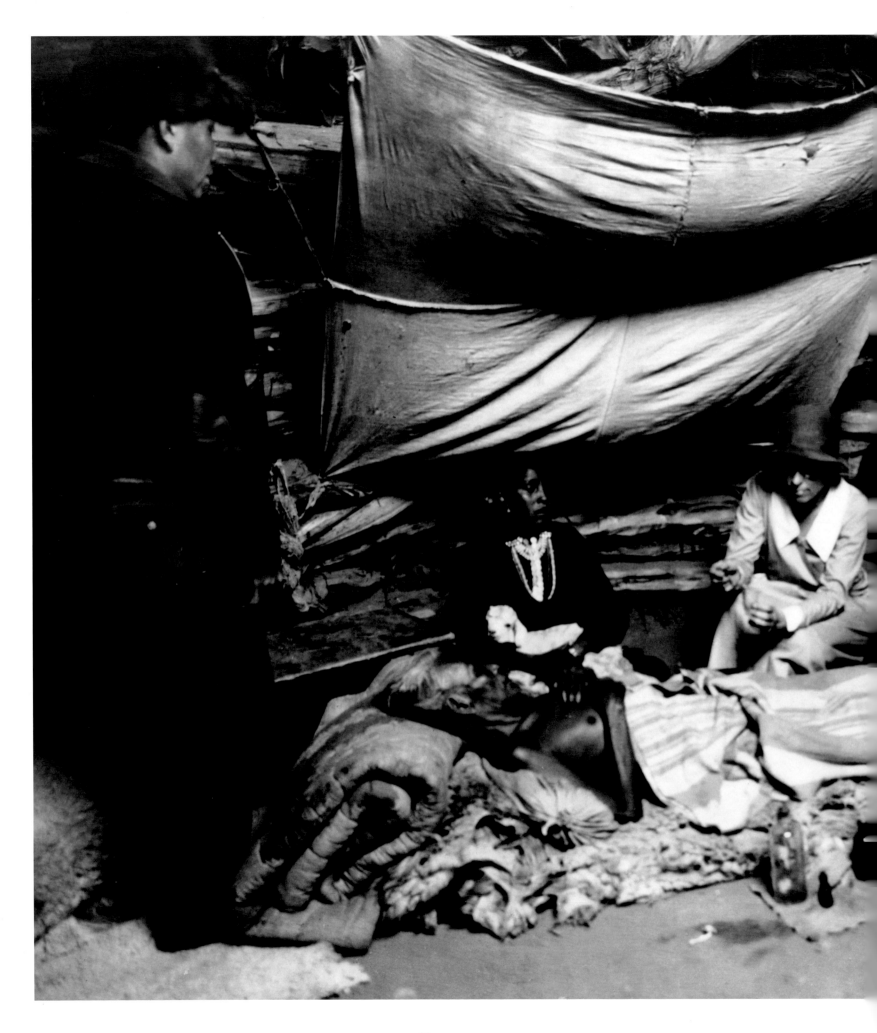

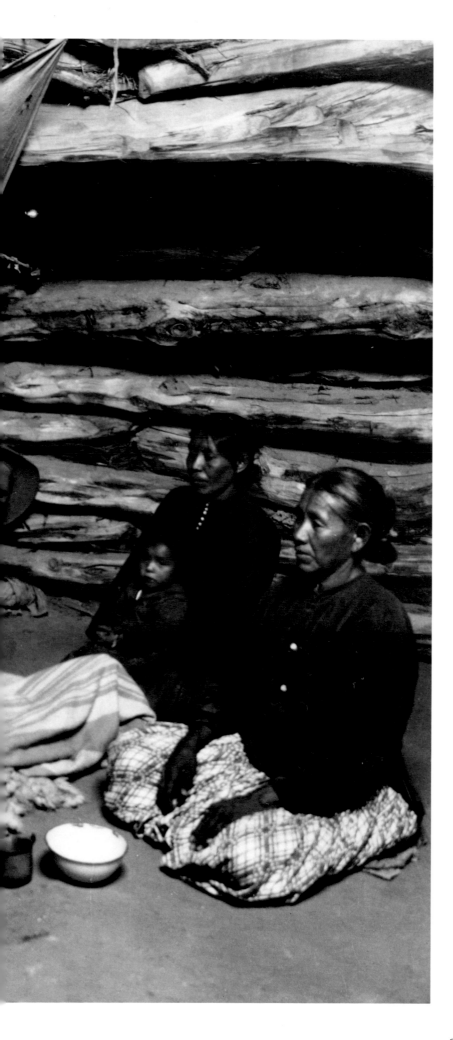

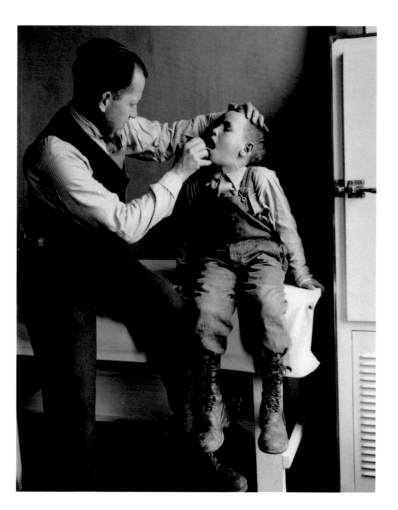

enced by the growing number of women in the field. Dramatic increases in the number of women in medical schools across the country (fifty-one percent of Michigan State and University of Massachusetts' graduating classes in 1992, to name just two examples) have changed the professional face of medicine. Regina Morantz, writing on the impact of women in medicine in *Sympathy and Science* (Oxford, 1985), asserted that "in medicine . . . a new appreciation has appeared for the traditionally 'female' qualities of nurturing and cooperation . . . with women physicians exhibiting a greater concern for patients' moral and emotional well-being." So as the century ends, the criticisms and issues of medicine not solved in the last century are being raised again with greater vehemence, as the determination of how, where, and to whom medicine is taught is undergoing major changes.

————

1932—*(left) Hardbelly's Hogan, Arizona. In the 1920s, with Native Americans largely confined to reservations in the West, the only hope for medical assistance was the visiting nurse. Photographed by Laura Gilpin.*

1938—*(above) There has always been a shortage of doctors in rural America, especially when times are hard. During the Depression, the people of Reedsville, West Virginia felt fortunate to get a physician. Photographed by Arthur Rothstein.*

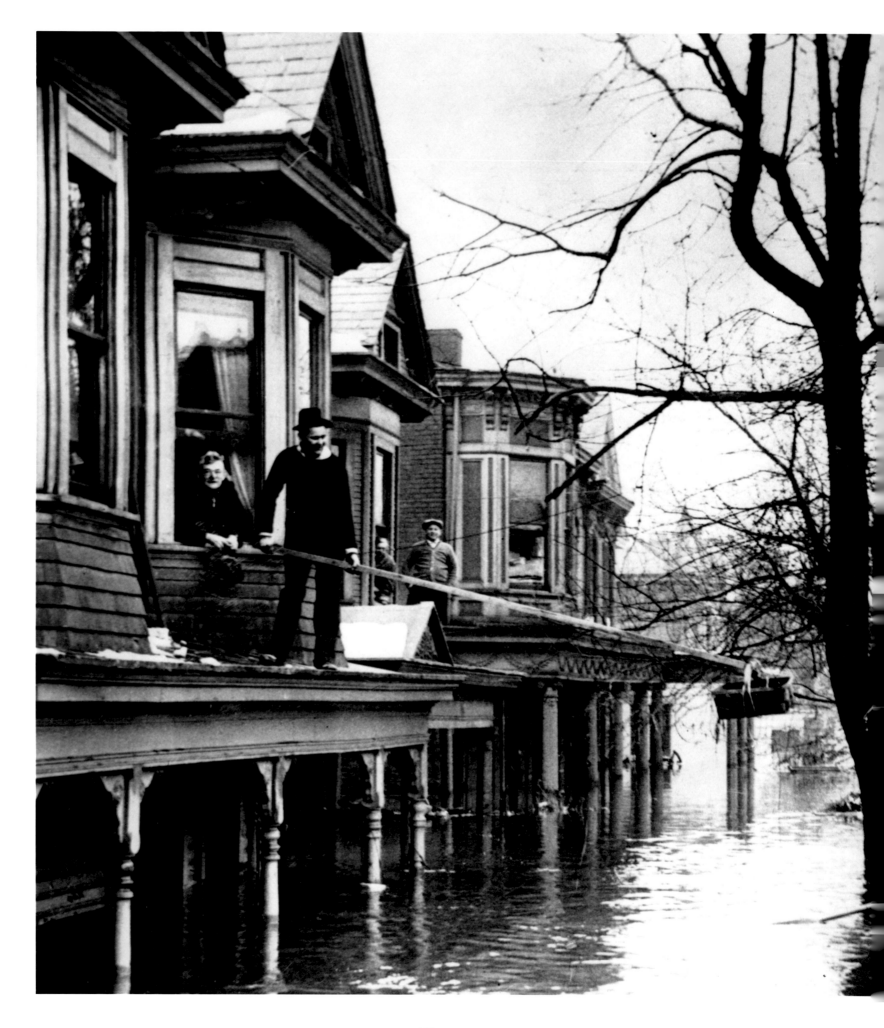

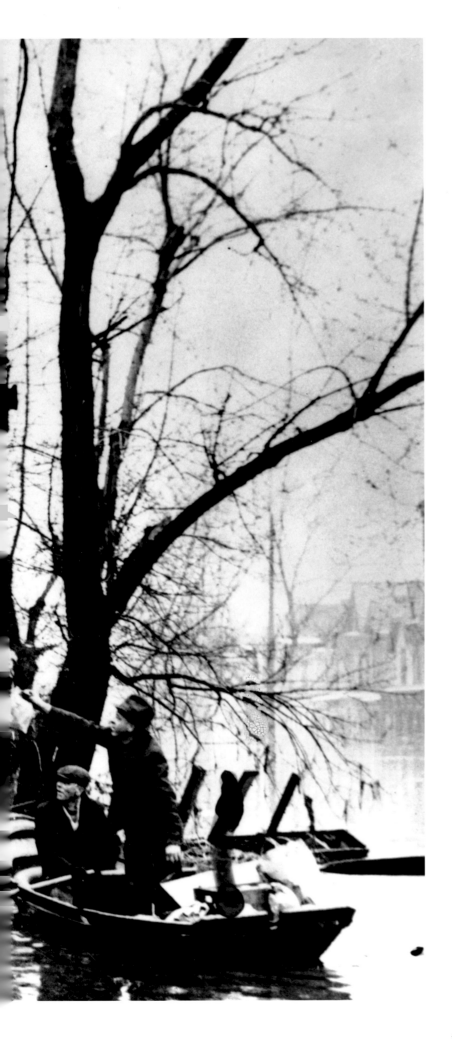

Nevertheless, throughout this century, there have been many doctors of every nationality who, without any evident prodding, turned away from money, home, and comfort to venture out to places and situations that would entail great risks and discomfort. They volunteered for war or set up shop in some tiny place where they were lucky if they could be paid through barter. They settled among the poor or devised ways to bring health care to their deprived patients, through a hospital ship or a clinic in a van, via rowboat or by prop plane.

As the war in the Persian Gulf got under way in 1991, the military poured in and so did the doctors. One group, known as the Médecins sans Frontières (MSF), is a French medical organization of swashbuckling, romantic reputation that operates under the slogan "Our duty is to interfere." Members of MSF go where they are needed, not necessarily where they are invited (in 1985 the organization was actually thrown out of Ethiopia), and are able to mobilize anywhere in the world within seventy-two hours. When the MSF began in the early seventies, it could not be sure of attracting enough doctors and nurses at low pay to make a go of it. But in the nineties, it had eight hundred professionals in its ranks, with doctors earning a regal $11,000 a year.

An American group called Flying Doctors chooses the most difficult locations in which to practice medicine. In a group expedition to northern Mexico, an X-ray technician, an orthopedist, a pediatrician, and a nurse packed up their skills and flew off in a small plane to one lone village to bring some measure of improved health to the people. They charge patients nothing for their services.

It is not just clinical doctors who act upon the urge to do good; some researchers also perform their work almost as if they were artists slaving away in an attic. Thailand's Dr. Khunying Tranakchit Harinasuta is credited with discovering that the time-honored treatment for malaria, chloroquine, was running into trouble as parasites developed a resistance to it. To prove her point, she traveled and studied throughout southeast Asia, often paying for the research out of her own pocket.

The sacrifices and bold contributions of individual doctors have inspired governments to embark on broader cooperative efforts to study and control illness. But work on the global scale we see today was slow in coming. A major program was launched in 1851 when twelve countries attended an International Sanitary Conference in Paris. Yet a truly worldwide organizational effort awaited the 1948 formation of the United Nations' World Health Organization

---

1936—The floods of Wheeling, West Virginia. Natural disasters frequently bring out the best in medicine, as heroic rescuers make it to the scene one way or another with doctors, nurses, and medical supplies.

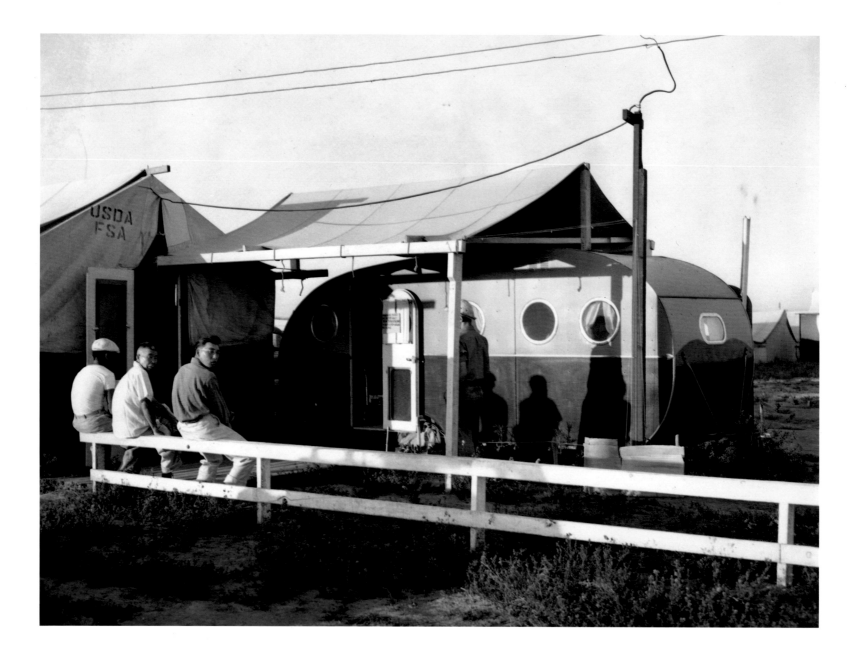

to monitor epidemiological and statistical information among more than one hundred fifty countries.

MEDICINE AT WAR

If ever there was any doubt that the devastation of war advances the cause of medicine, the conflagrations of the last century prove the point. One hundred years of war brought a sharpened awareness of the need for dramatically improved medicine and for a heightened ability to respond to emergencies vigorously enough to save lives. The buildup of military defenses mandated a corresponding response from medical schools, nursing services, and public health programs. With each conflict, the challenges shifted.

In the words of the Union Surgeon General, the American Civil War was fought "at the end of the medical middle ages," when physicians amputated limbs only to lose patients to infection. The doctors were helpless in the face of diseases that *(continued on page 110)*

1942—*(above) Even during the horrors of Japanese-American internment in the United States, medical care was made available, as at this mobile unit in Nyssa, Oregon. Photographed by Russell Lee.*

1939—*(opposite) In a nation that increasingly saw quality health care as a right, rural doctors in a southwest clinic introduced allergy testing to patients, both young and old. Photographed by Hansel Mieth.*

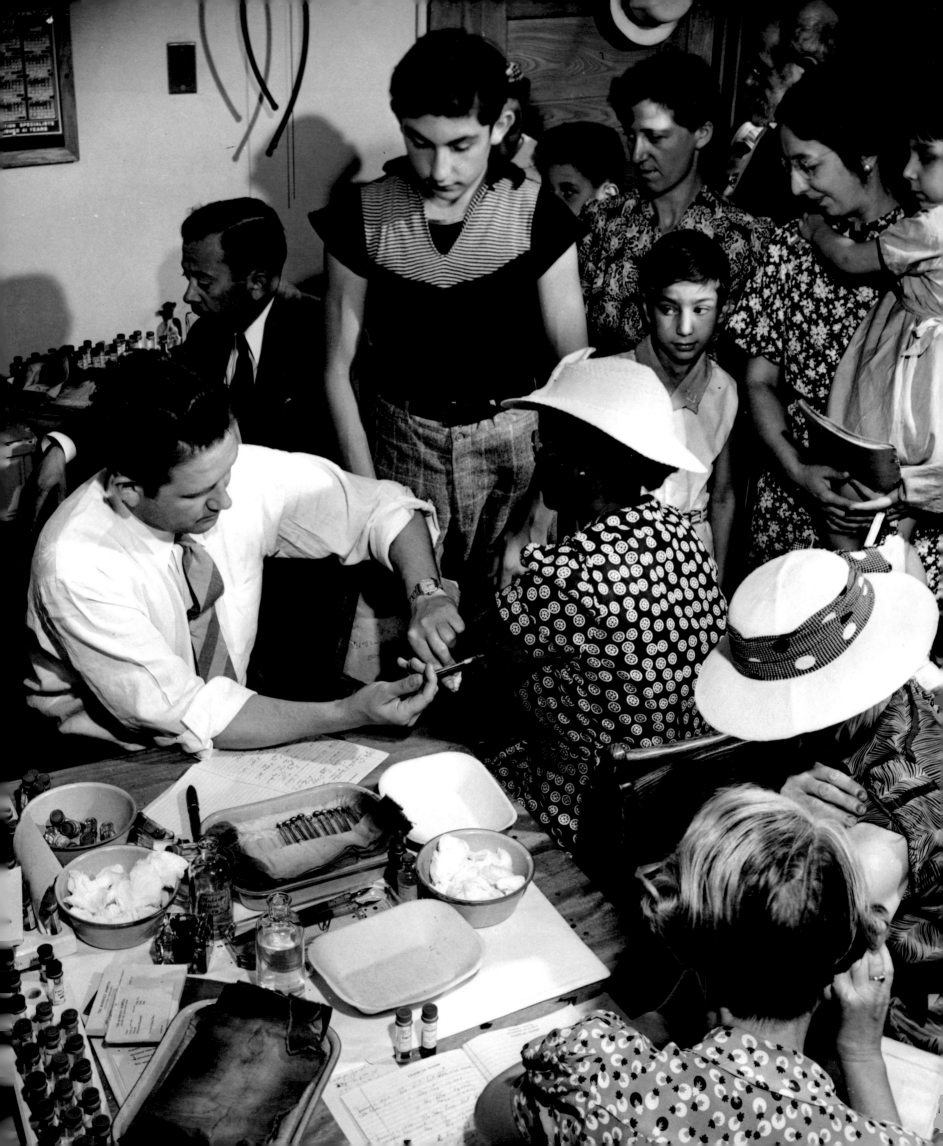

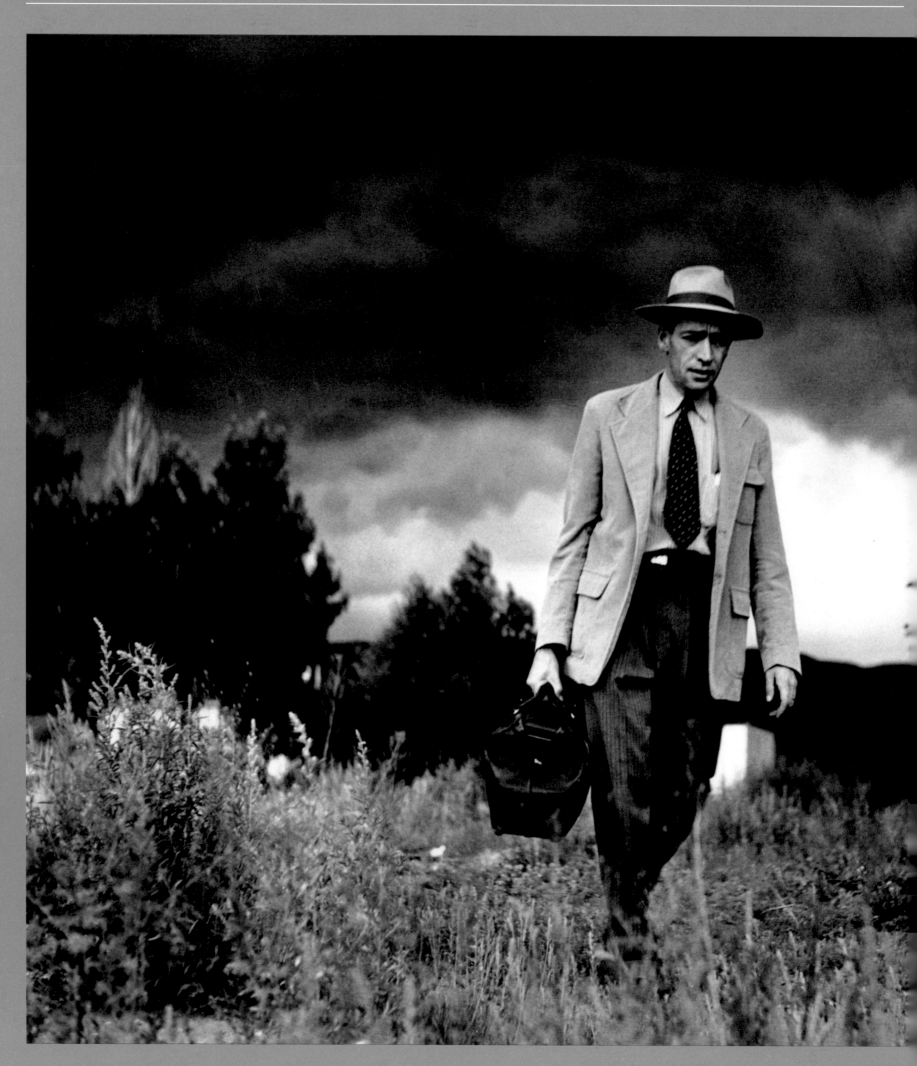

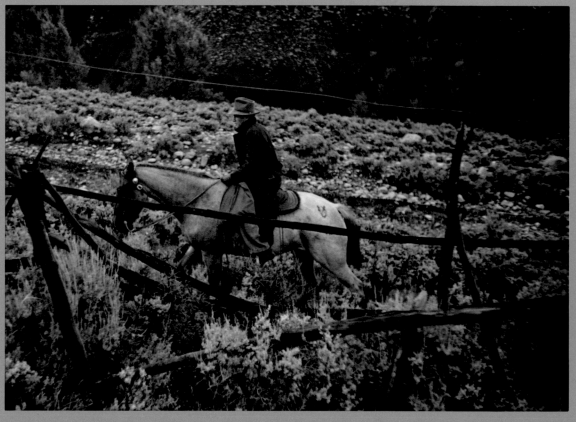

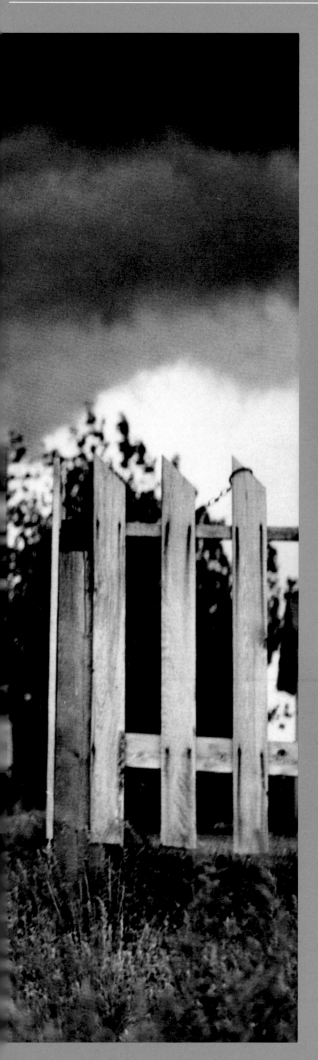

A Day in the Life of a Country Doctor

1948—*Life* Magazine sent W. E. Smith to Kremmling, Colorado, to photograph a country doctor at work. Smith met and befriended Dr. Ernest Ceriani. "Country Doctor" was a breakthrough for Smith and for photojournalism. Avoiding potential cliches, Smith created an earnest, empathetic portrait of an American folk hero. Dr. Ceriani was on call day and night, and so was Smith. He captured the doctor delivering babies, comforting patients, and binding wounds, enlarging his portrait with rare and private moments of relaxation—Ceriani riding horseback, or catching a cup of coffee. In Smith's own words, "I spent four weeks living with him. I made very few pictures at first. I mainly tried to learn what made the doctor tick, what his personality was, how he worked and what the surroundings were.

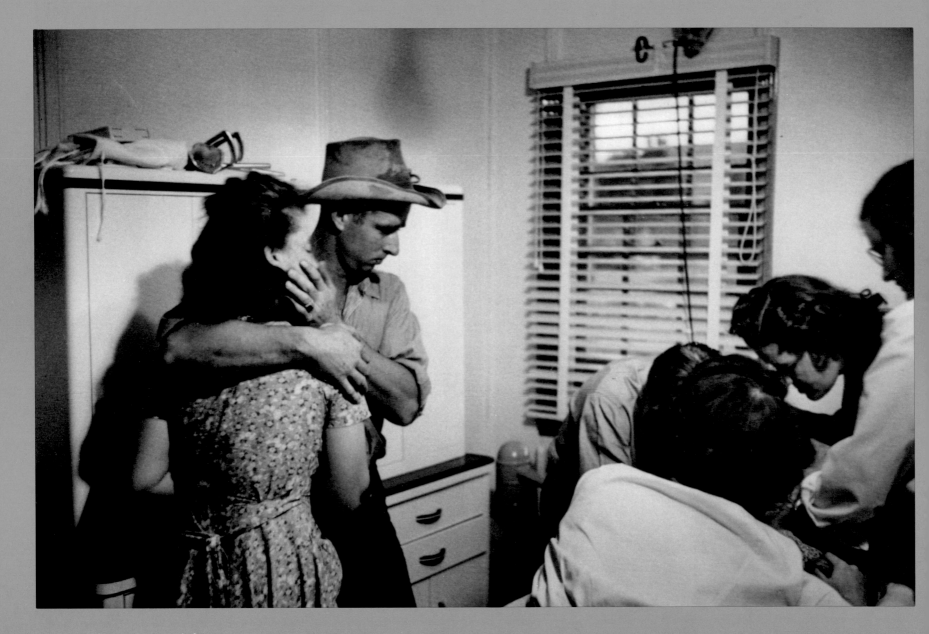

I had to wait for actuality instead of setting up poses. I simply faded into wallpaper and waited. By fading, by being in the background, I was able to catch expressions and emotions. I moved quickly and didn't open my mouth. The doctor was terrific—a grand fellow, which leads me to say that with any long story you have to be compatible with your subject, as I was with him. I reserve my temperament for home and the darkroom." Within the "Country Doctor" essay, Smith told the story of two-and-a-half-year-old Lee Marie Wheatly. Dr. Ceriani was called in to perform emergency surgery after the young girl was kicked in the head by a horse *(above and opposite)*. Ceriani was sure she would lose an eye, and attempted to find a way to gently tell her parents. At the end of a long day, Ceriani relaxed with a cup of coffee *(right)*.

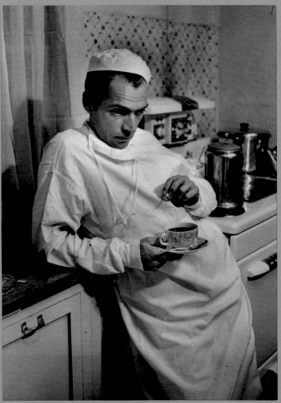

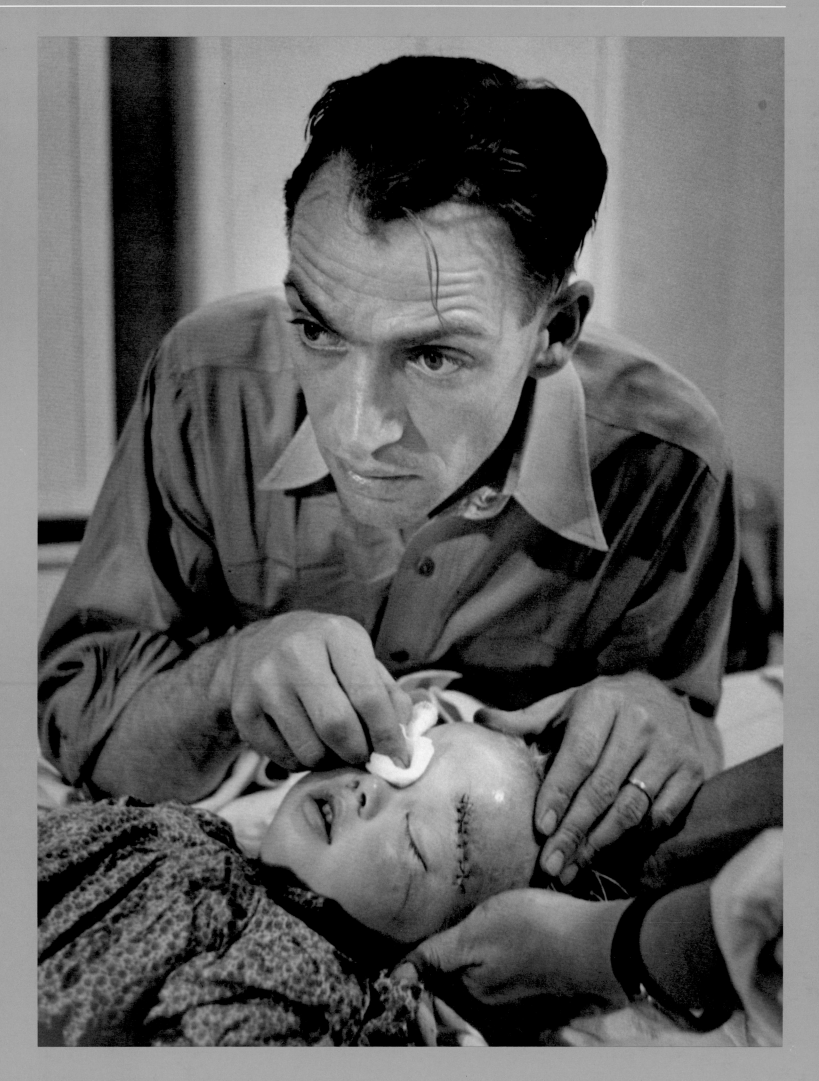

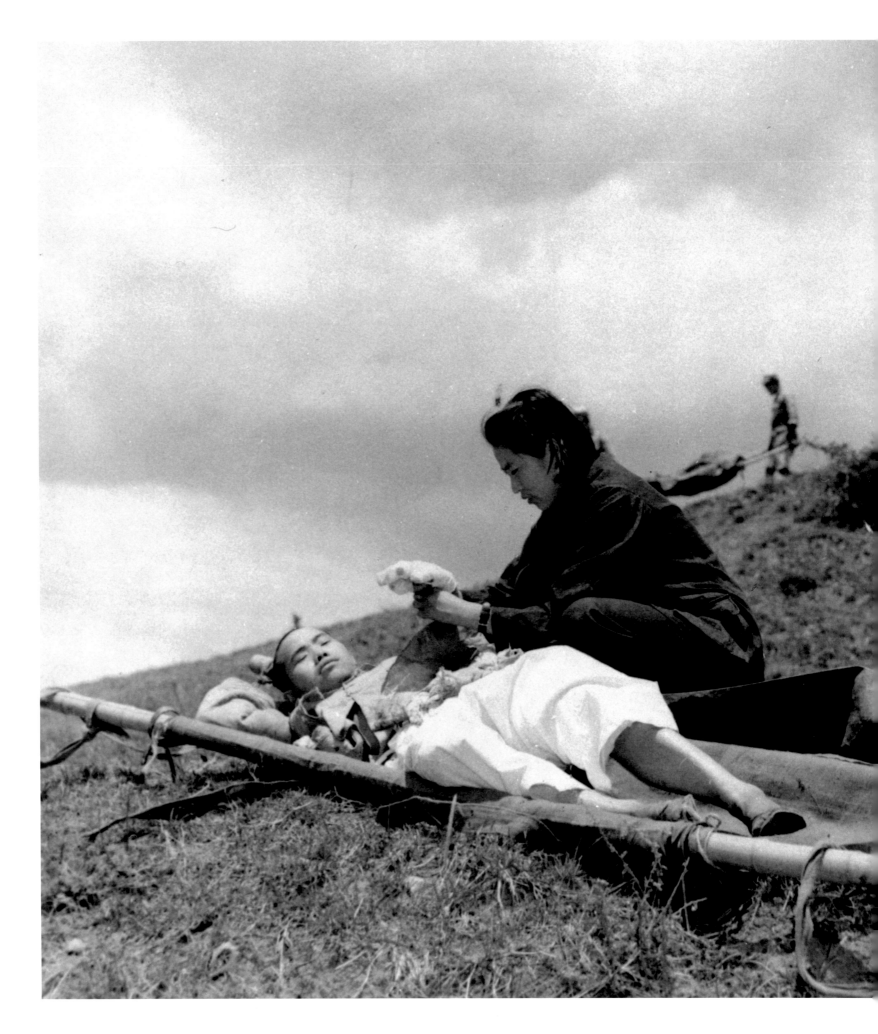

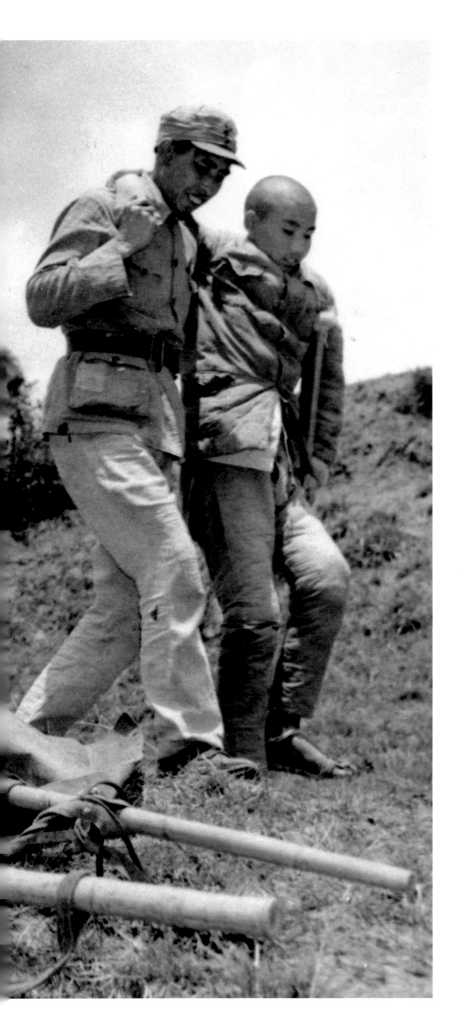

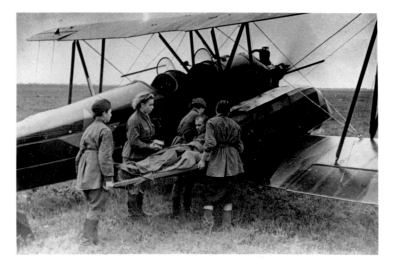

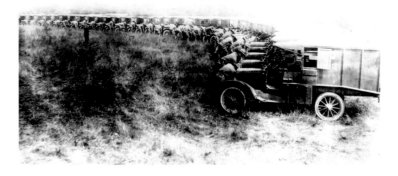

Circa 1942—*(above top) Transportation of the wounded, greatly improved by the airplane, was a key to better medical care in World War II.*

1917—*(above) In World War I, the battlefield ambulance had a starring role, as it whisked the wounded to the hospital.*

Circa 1940—*(left) With their long tradition of wartime service, nurses expect to work on the front lines, as this one is doing, in China, during World War II.*

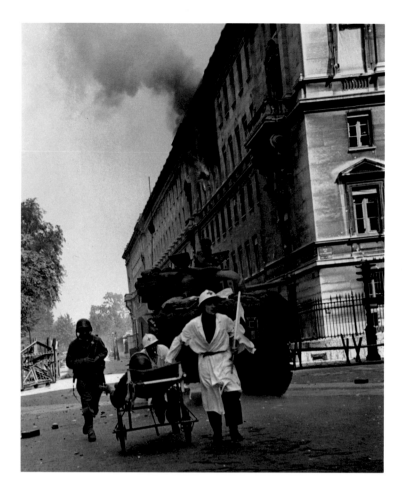

raced through their wards. By the time of World War I, the depredations of submarine warfare, air assault, and trench warfare prompted a level of resourcefulness in medical response unparalleled in history. Thanks to pioneering efforts by Florence Nightingale in the Crimean War and Clara Barton in the Civil War, World War I was the first conflict in which nurses had professional training, and they quickly made themselves indispensable. Hospitalization was seen as the largest and most difficult problem both armies faced, and the front-line station, the field hospital, and the base hospital evolved to meet the need. It was a baptism of blood for medicine, culminating in the horrors of a war-born pandemic of influenza that swept the world at the end of 1918.

By World War II, medicine could be *(continued on page 115)*

───────

1944—*(above) It's near the end of the war in Paris, but the wounded keep coming. Photographed by Robert Capa.*

1918—*(right) American soldiers wounded during the first day's fighting in the Argonne forest wait in a bombed-out church until they can be moved to the rear for treatment. The day's losses were light compared with the rest of the campaign, but transporting the wounded was difficult: the roads through the area had been torn up by four years of shellfire, and steady rains meant that ambulances had to make their way over muddy ground to reach evacuation hospitals.*

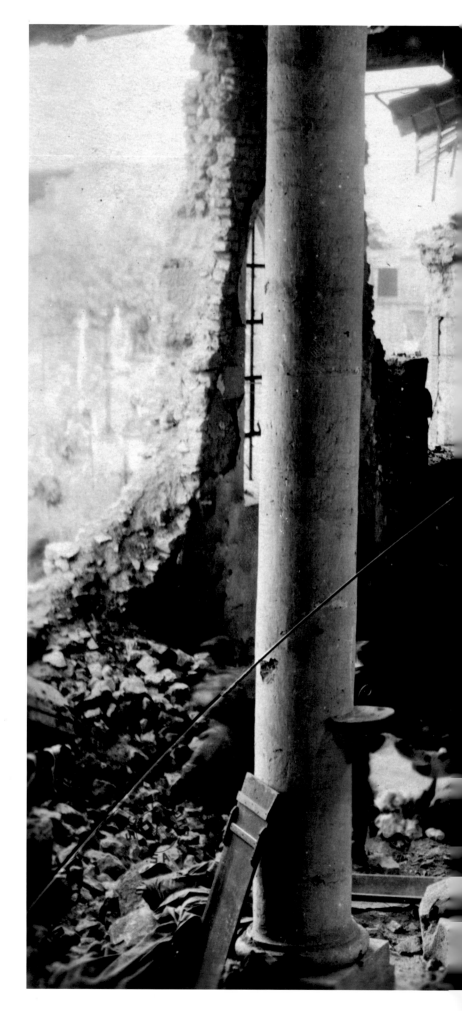

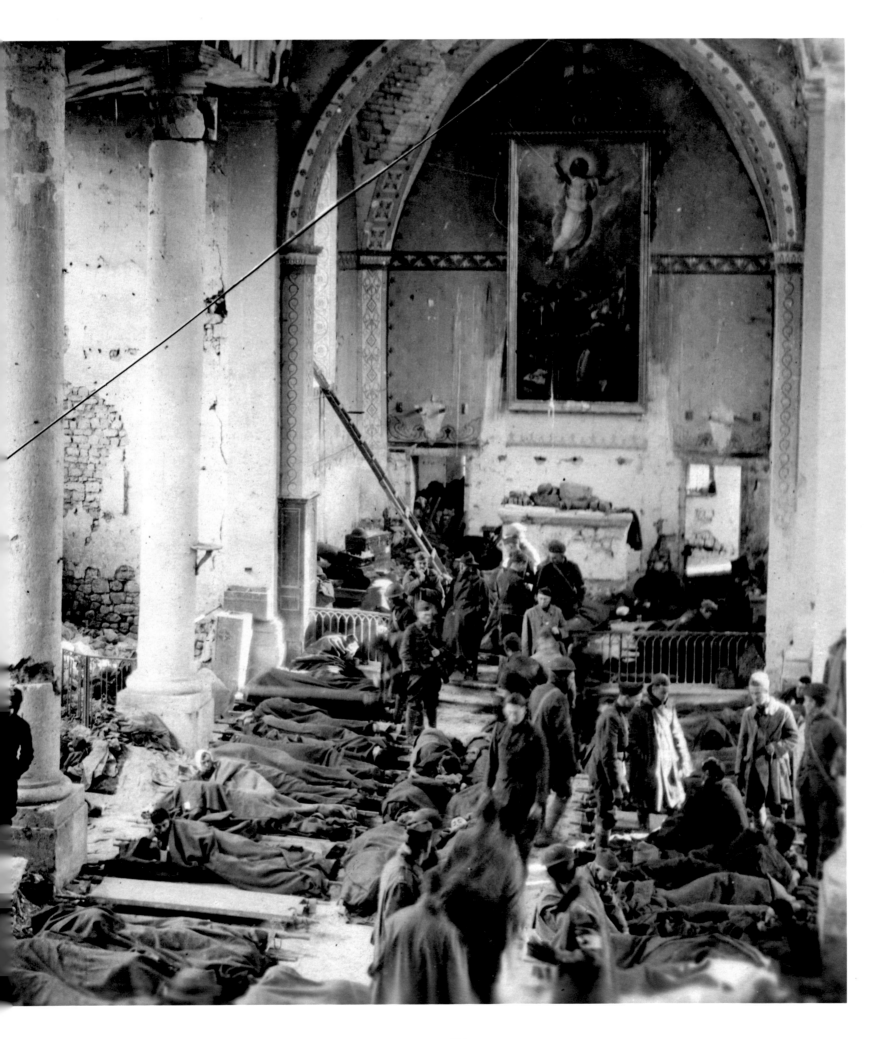

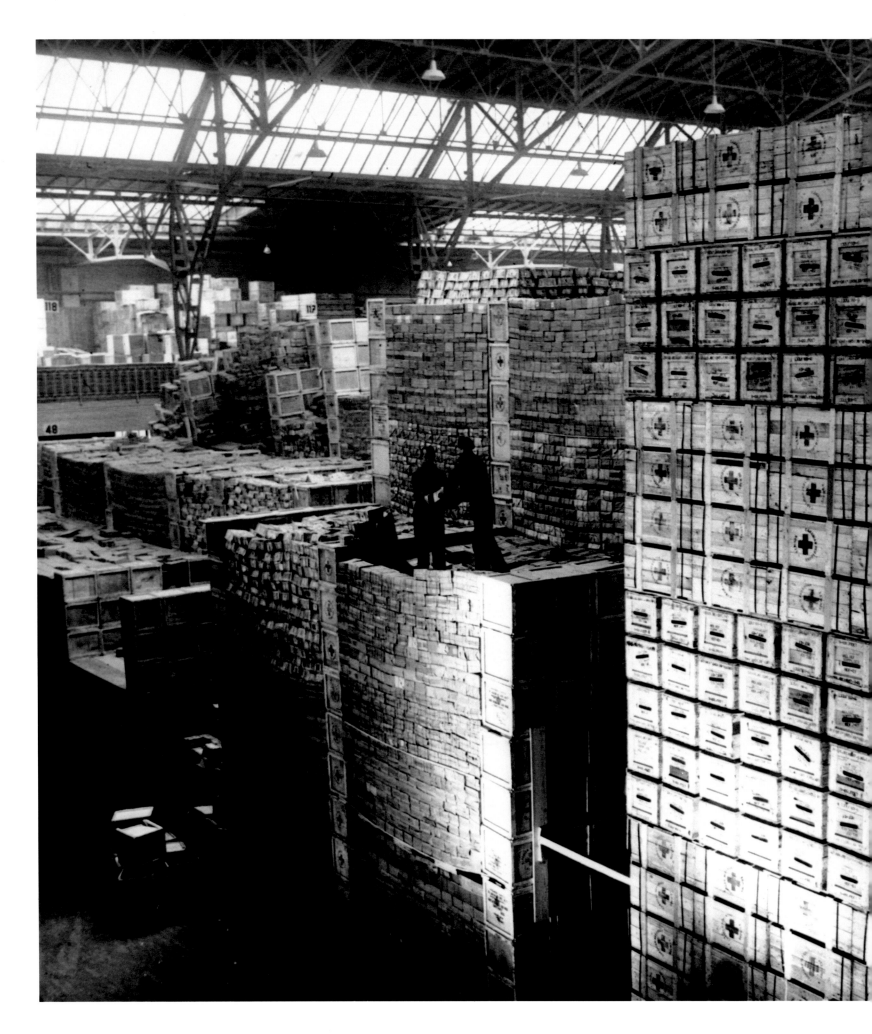

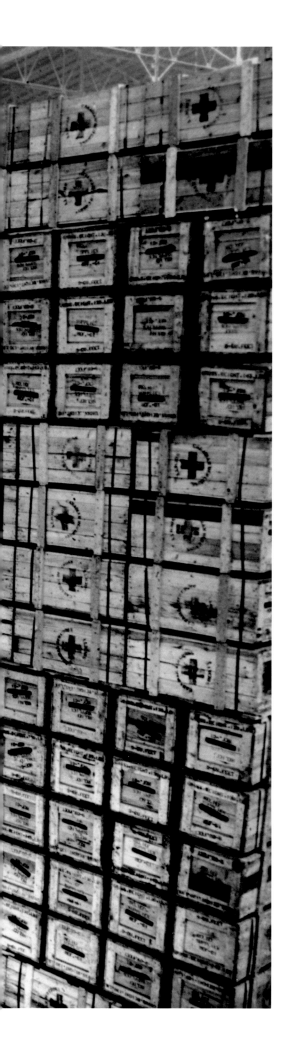

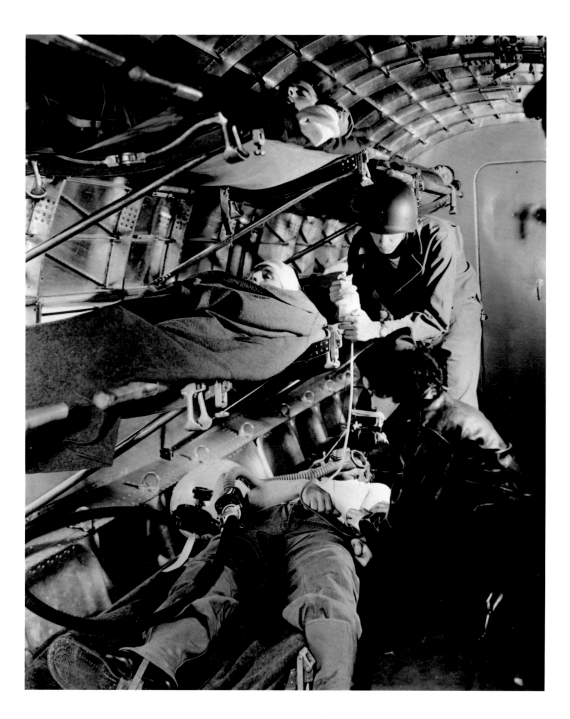

Circa 1942—*(left) In the medical care of World War II soldiers, the Red Cross played an enormous role around the world. Here, packages of food and clothing are piled high in Geneva awaiting shipment through the international committee of the organization.*

Circa 1942—*(above) World War II: during wartime, even the hull of a plane became an emergency-care station for the wounded and the dying. The demand for plasma was tremendous, and blood-collection centers were opened all across the United States.*

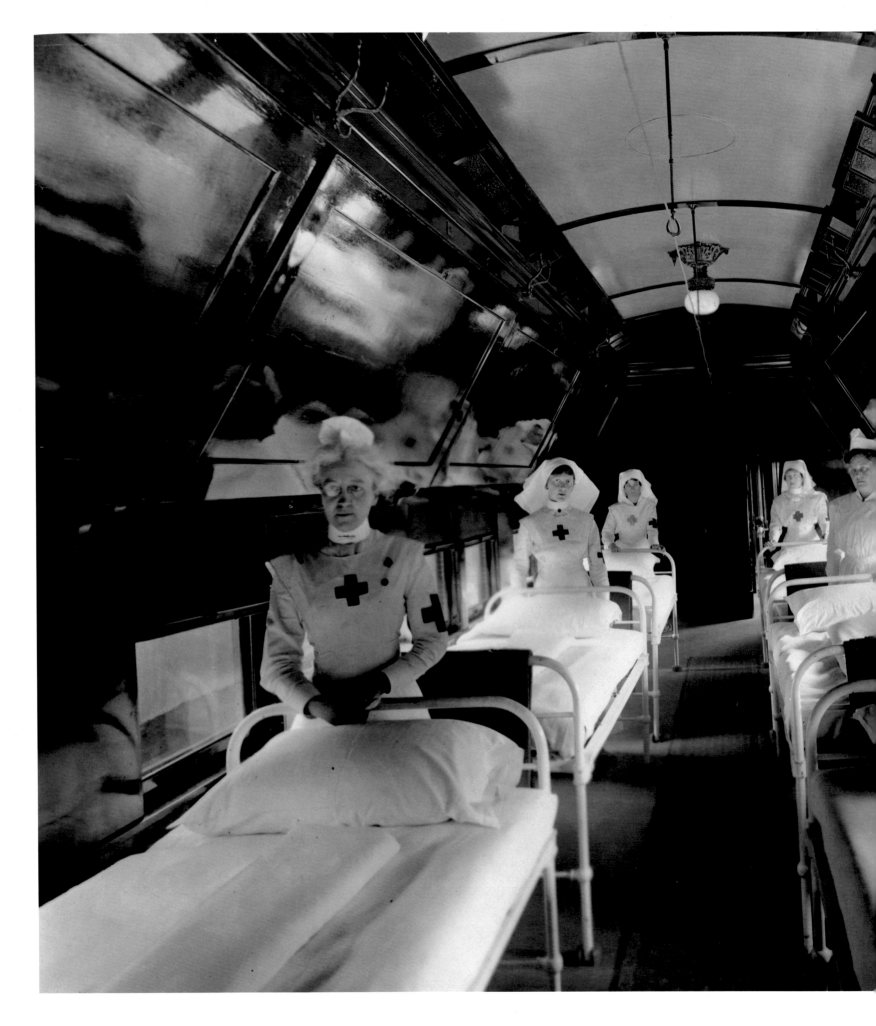

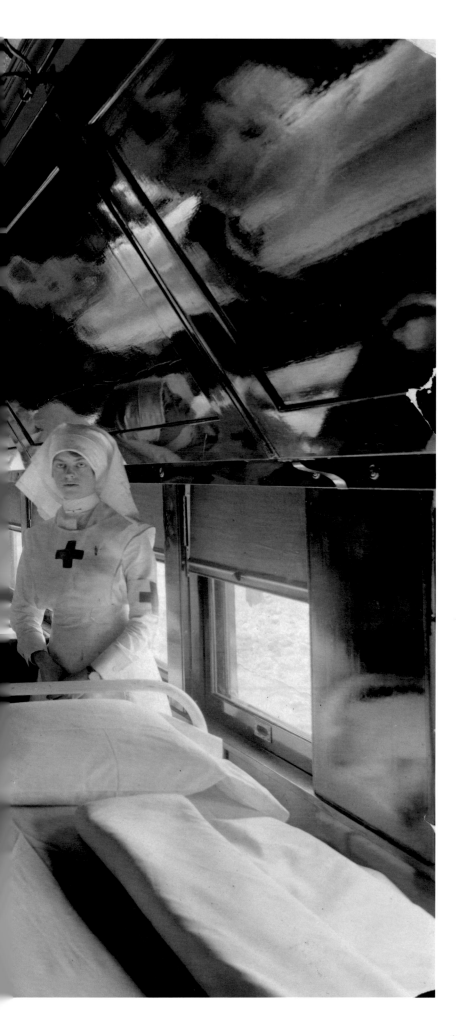

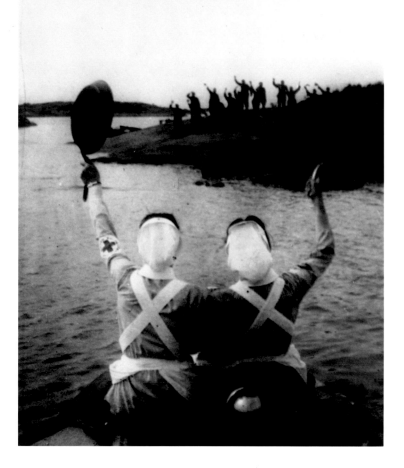

mobilized to meet the many calamities of battle. The heroism of doctors and nurses was a given. The tools of military medicine had expanded exponentially, to include sulfa drugs, penicillin, new developments in antimalarial therapy, and the ready availability of blood and blood derivatives. Transport by air, ship, or train was available to carry the wounded, and nursing's key role was firmly defined. Military medicine's emphasis on ever-greater speed is regarded as the single greatest factor in keeping the mortality rate lower in World War II than in World War I. In Korea, the Mobile Army Surgical Hospitals (better known as MASH) were clearing stations to stabilize the severely wounded before sending them to the rear for care. By the time of the long-running conflagration in Vietnam, where no front lines existed in the traditional sense, helicopters became the rescuing angels, descending from the sky to whisk the wounded away from the fight and toward help at base hospitals far from the front lines. *(continued on page 121)*

———

Circa 1930—*(left) Demonstrating inventiveness in creating mobile health care in time of need, the Canadian Pacific Railway committed some of its cars to serve as wards. Here nurses stand at the ready.*

Circa 1940—*(above) Nurses of the German Red Cross.*

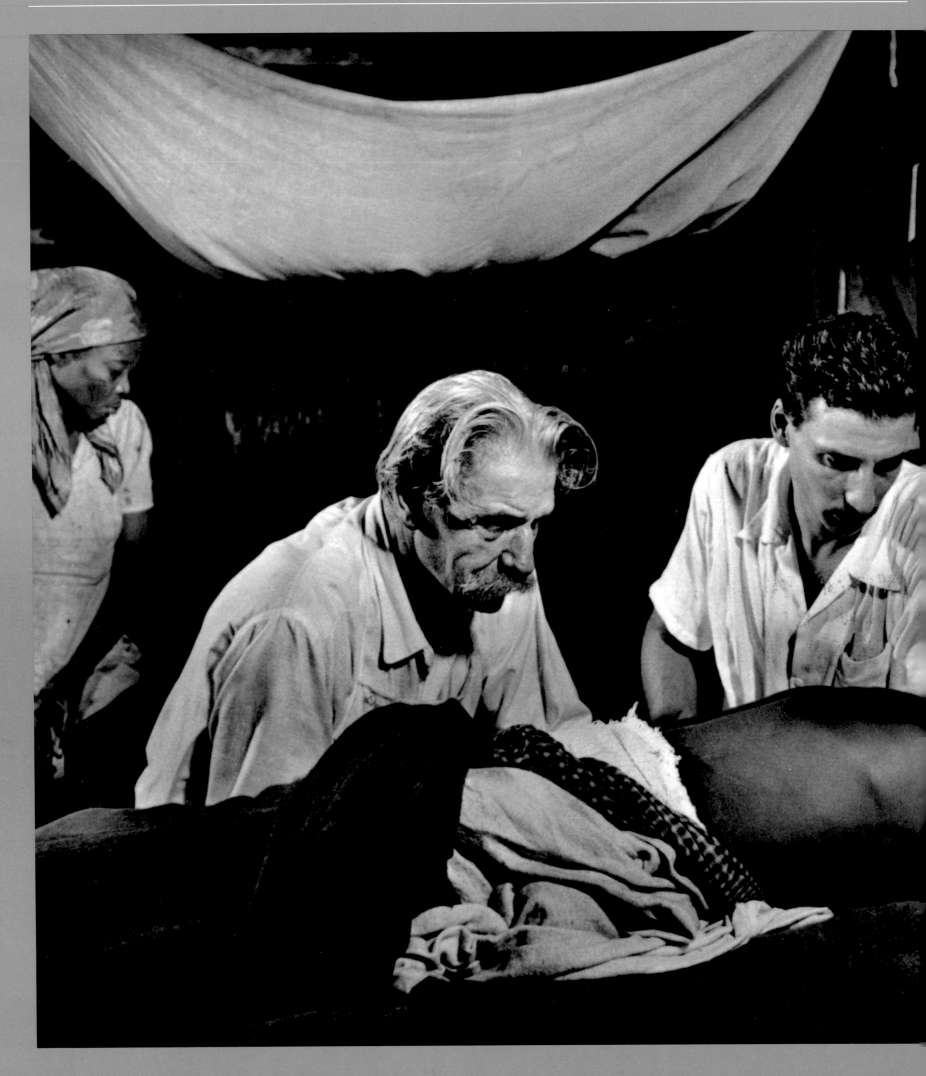

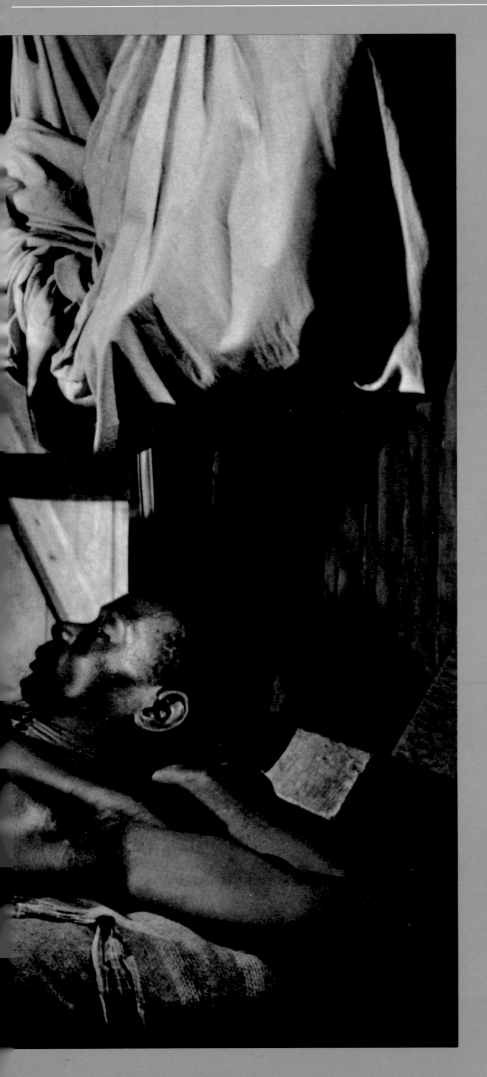

On the Edge of Civilization

Albert Schweitzer (1875-1965) was a theologian and a musician and brilliant at both. But it was his work as a medical missionary that brought Schweitzer's name and his values to the attention of the entire world. After receiving his medical doctorate at the University of Strasbourg, he established a hospital at Lambaréné, Gabon, in 1913. Except for extensive fund-raising trips, he remained in Gabon thereafter, expanding the medical facilities. Winner of the 1952 Nobel Peace Prize for his efforts to create "a brotherhood of nations," he contributed the prize money to building a village for lepers. The photographs here, like those of the country doctor *(pages 104-107)*, are by W. E. Smith for *Life*.

Although the photographs are a triumph of Smith's artistry, the assignment ended on a sour note when the photographer and the magazine disagreed over how many would be published—and Smith resigned. From the beginning, Smith was passionately involved in the assignment: he regarded Schweitzer with a mixture of respect, awe, and envy. Smith later described his visit to Schweitzer this way: "The visitor, unprepared, will even have difficulty in trying to determine the nature of the place: whether it is an African village, a game preserve, or a medical hospital. Actually, it is the sum of the three. It is a wisdom, a philosophy, a total meaning uniquely its own."

1954—*(left)* Schweitzer with patient at the Lambaréné hospital in Gabon.

1954—*(right)* The streets of Lamberéné, Gabon. Schweitzer carries the tool of his trade, his stethoscope, on route to visit a patient *(opposite, right)*. A patient receives a draught of medicine from one of the doctor's assistants *(opposite, far right)*. Surgery at the make-shift hospital *(opposite, below)*. Schweitzer's philosophy was known for its oracular brevity. "Ethics are pity," he said, adding "All life is suffering." But, as he quickly confided to a visitor, there was no time for discussion, "for we are too busy fighting pain."

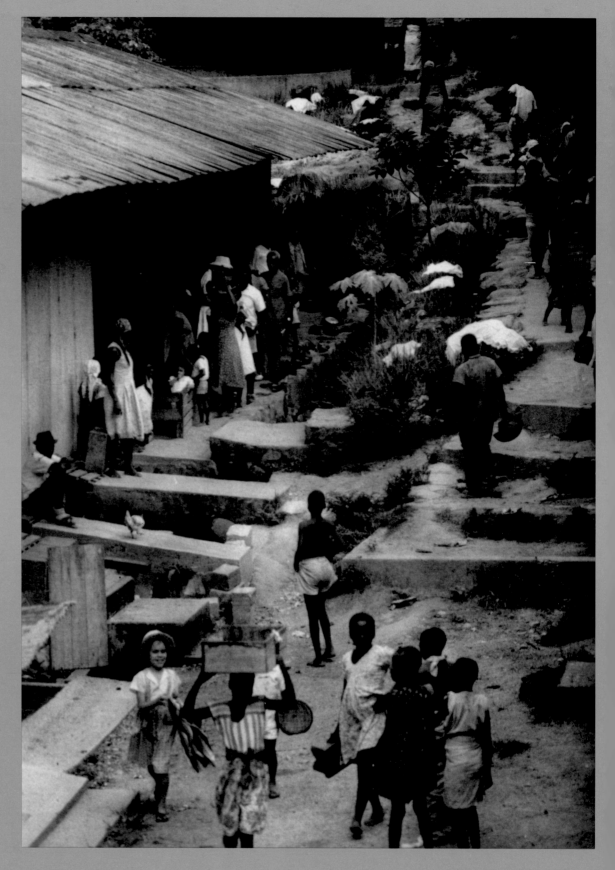

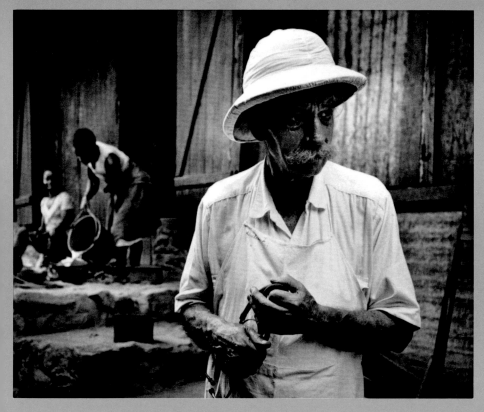

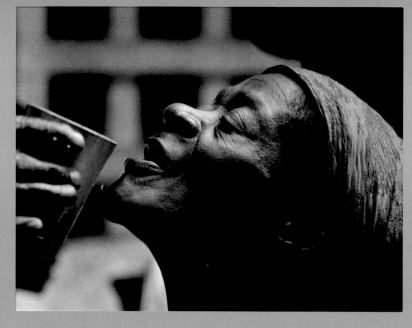

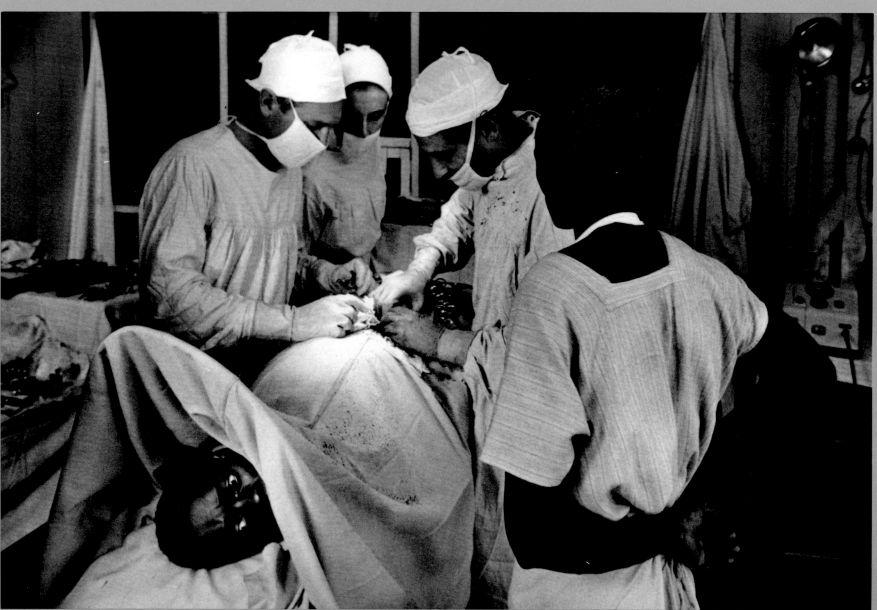

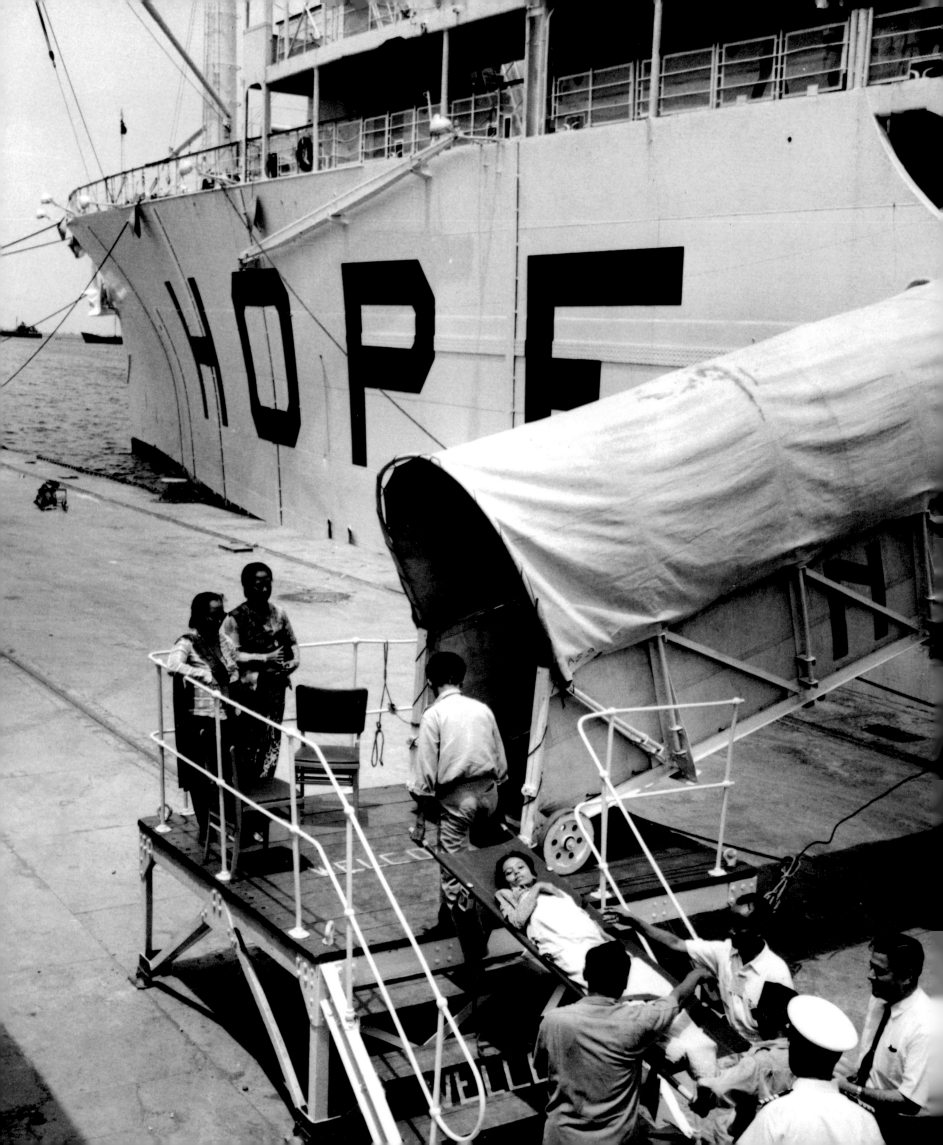

1961—(opposite) The 15,000-ton ship originally called Consolation was renamed Hope and plunged into service in 1960 as the world's first peacetime hospital ship. Cruising the world, it brought modern health care wherever there was a coastline and a need. Photographed by John Dominus.

1980—(right) In the hallowed tradition of the caregiver as exemplar of goodness, Mother Teresa set a sterling example of tending to the poor around the world. She was born Agnes Gonxha Bojaxhiu in 1910 in Skopje, Yugoslavia, entered the Loreto Convent, and then left it for the teeming streets and the poorest of the poor. Now her Missionaries of Charity—the nurse shown here is a member of one of those organizations—number 158 houses worldwide, with 2,500 nuns and 10,000 lay volunteers caring for unwed mothers, lepers, the retarded, the dying, and the insane. "We must," Mother Teresa says, "do our work as if everything depends on us—then leave the rest to God." Photographed by Mary Ellen Mark.

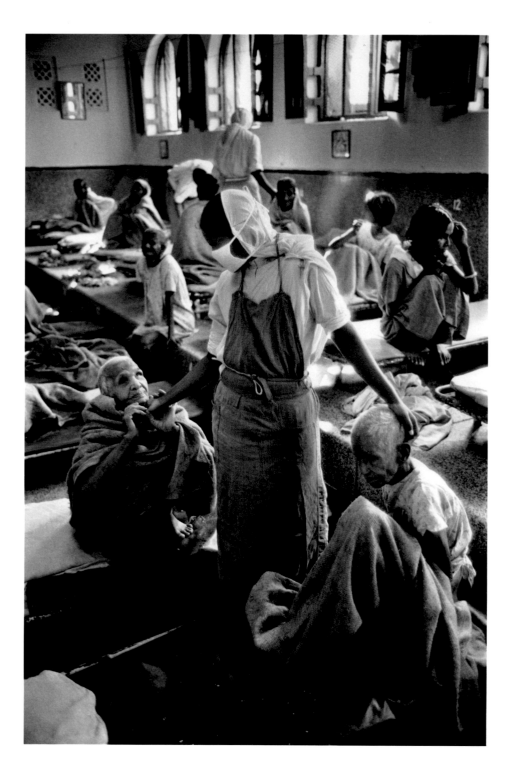

One of the most dramatic, altruistic undertakings of twentieth-century medicine was Project Hope, which sent the world's first peacetime hospital ship on eleven different world voyages, bringing medicine to destinations as diverse as Peru and Vietnam. The ship they dubbed the *Hope* had been the *Consolation*—15,000 tons and none too spiffy, already fifteen years old and the veteran of two wars. The project was begun by a Washington cardiologist, Bill Walsh, who once told an interviewer that the idea went "back to my days as a medical officer on a destroyer in the South Pacific during World War II. It was pretty clear to me as a young

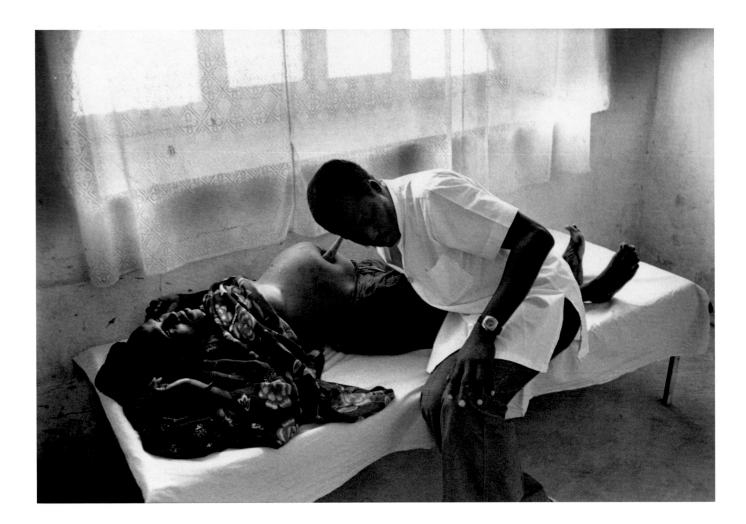

physician that there was no health care in that part of the world. I decided if I ever got a chance, I'd do something about it." Once Project Hope was under way, it employed only doctors who agreed to work purely as volunteers, receiving air fare to and from the ship as their stipend, while the rest of the staff got $300 a month. If ever one doubted that a goodly number of contemporary doctors and nurses are ready to forgo riches, the experience of Project Hope is instructive. Two thousand nurses volunteered to fill twenty-two slots as the ship brought cancer screening to Ceylon, nurse training to Guyana, and heart surgery to Poland. Although the project continued as a landbased organization afterward, the ship's adventure in health care lasted only fourteen years, from 1960 to 1974, on the high seas.

As today's doctors and nurses travel the globe, invariably they come to realize that cures are not everything. These days prevention has taken on new importance everywhere—the avid attention to diet that is now part of life in the developed world is a prime example—but it is an even more crucial element of medicine's goal in the Third World. There, forty thousand children die each day, mostly from dehydration and starvation. Battles won in industrialized nations at the beginning of the century are still being fought in these poorer countries. The need for *(continued on page 128)*

1979—*(above) A country doctor brings prenatal care to a woman in Chad. Photographed by Raymond Depardon.*

1978—*(right) A woman belonging to the Ogandan tribe in Ethiopia is vaccinated with a few quick jabs to protect her against smallpox. Unlike many diseases, the smallpox virus has no known reservoir other than man. Transmission normally occurs from personal contact, and a victim rarely infects more than five others. The disease spreads slowly and, in scarring its survivors, leaves visible evidence that it was present. Photographed by Marion Kaplan.*

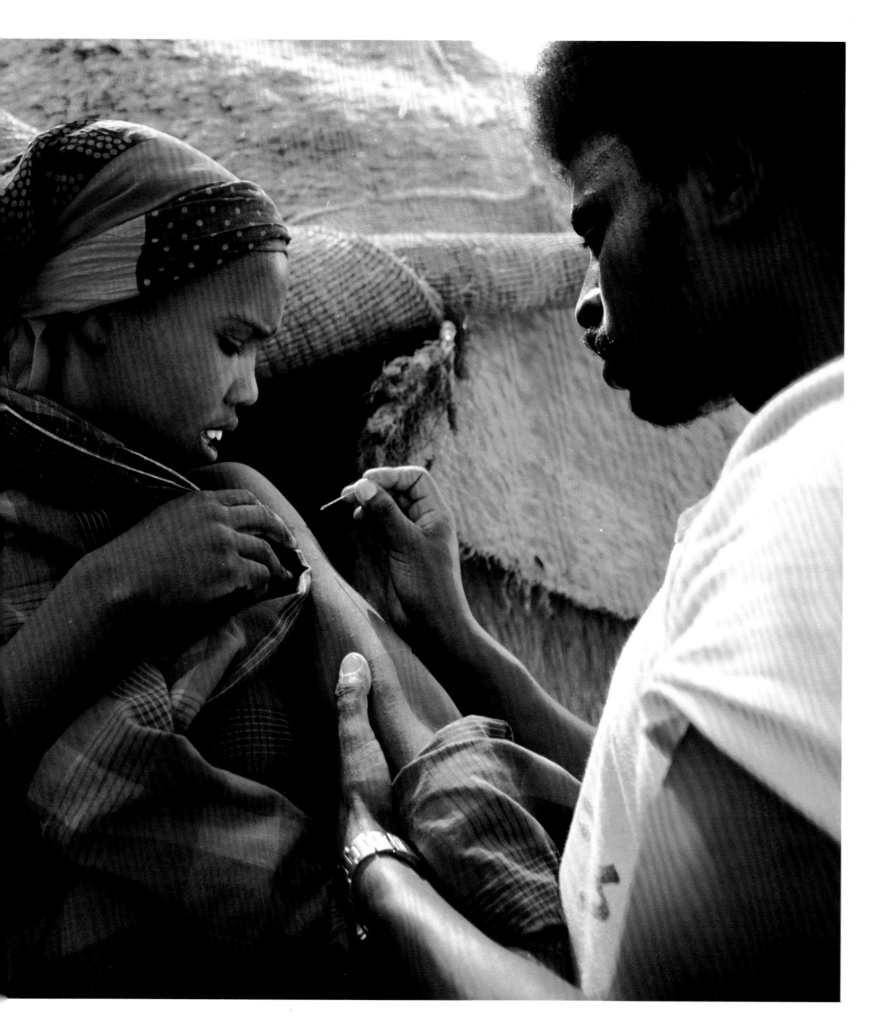

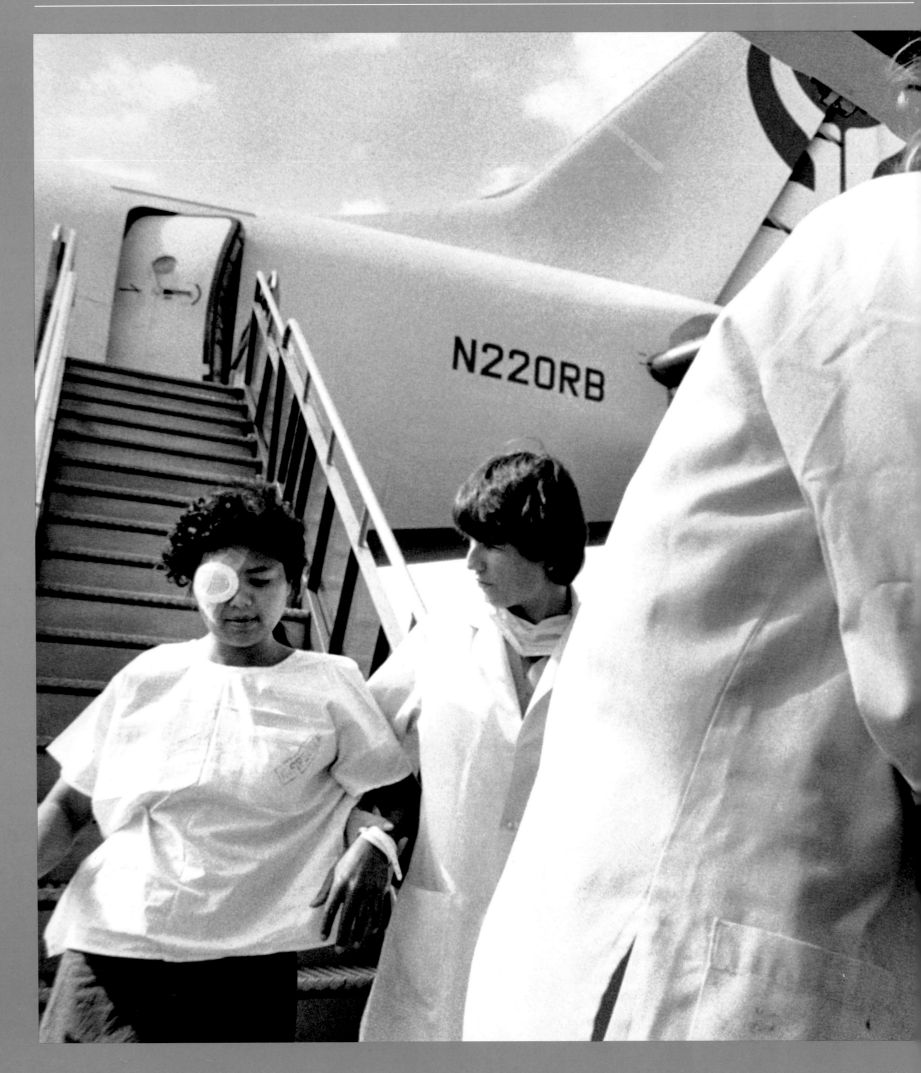

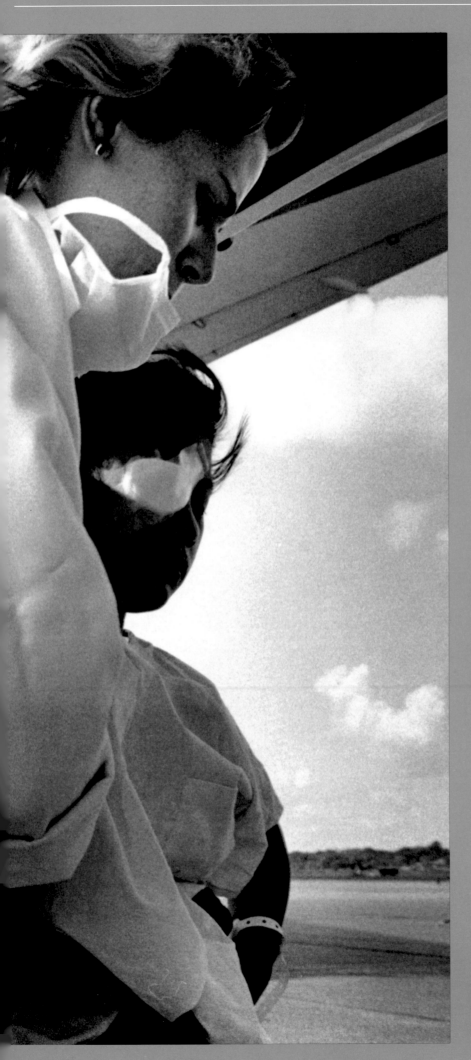

The Hospital with Wings

1991—Despite the advances of modern medicine, blindness—especially in much of the developing world—remains a scourge of mankind. Aiming to prevent blindness where it can and correcting other vision problems as well, Project Orbis and its DC-8 flying hospital have traversed the globe.

On one mission *(left)*, the team of volunteer doctors and nurses—led by Orbis' president, Oliver Foot—spent three weeks teaching, operating, lecturing, and getting to know their Burmese counterparts at the Yangon Eye, Ear, Nose, and Throat Hospital. Orbis even arranged for corneas by the boxful to be shipped to the hospital *(below)*. There, the organization's doctors paid particular attention to the children *(below bottom)*, among them, youngsters with crossed eyes hoping for surgery from specialist Dr. Black.

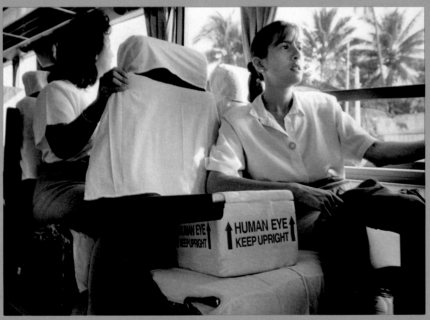

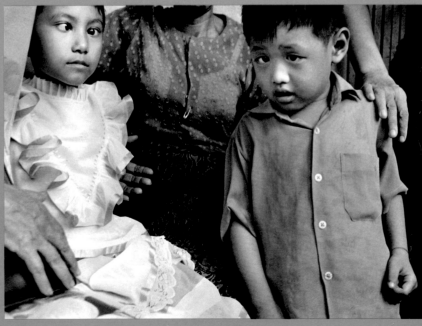

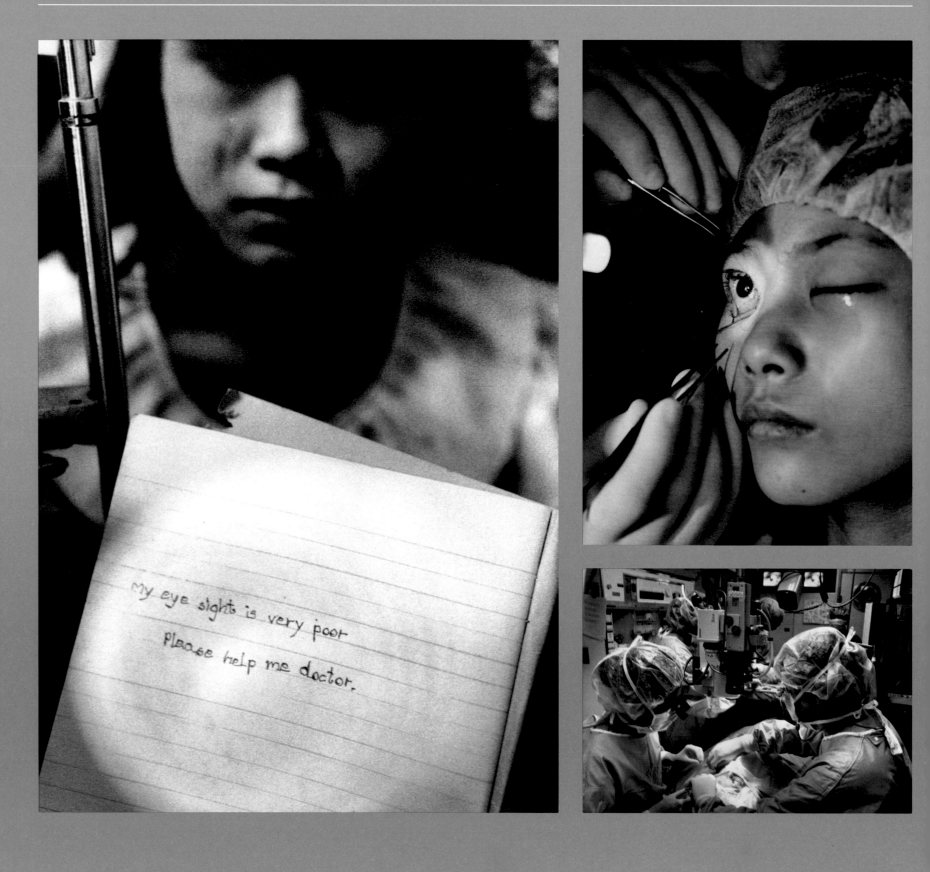

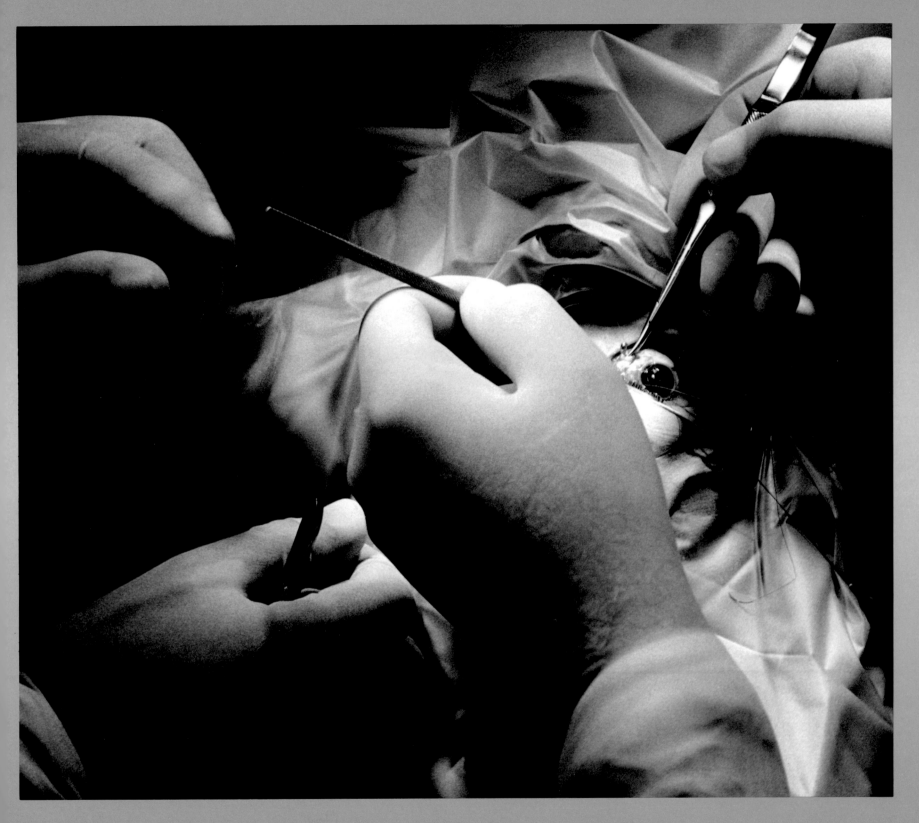

The Orbis doctors confronted one case that certainly seemed hopeless: Kin Than Dar Soe, a sixteen-year-old girl, had come into the clinic with milky eyes that appeared to be completely clouded over, the result of her mother's malaria during pregnancy. The physicians examined her and concluded that she was blind. Her mother denied it. If she was blind, how could she still write words on paper, as she always did? But surely the mother was deluding herself, the doctors told each other. Then Kin took pen in hand, bent over a sheet of paper, her eyelashes so close they brushed it, and began to write. It was an astonishing moment. She did have some sight left and could use it. The girl immediately became a candidate for remedial surgery (opposite left and top right).

Inside the Orbis DC-8 operating room, Dr. Black is assisted by Burmese surgeon Mae Win during one of the many operations to alleviate crossed eyes. The microphones attached to the surgeons' masks enable the doctors to discuss procedures with their colleagues in the classrooms (opposite, bottom right). Dr. Black sutures the muscle back to the eyeball of twelve-year-old Yin Mkon Nwe, correcting a cross-eyed condition (above).

At the end of the organization's three-week stay in Burma, Orbis had performed almost sixty different operations, assisted by local doctors.
Photographed by Misha Erwitt.

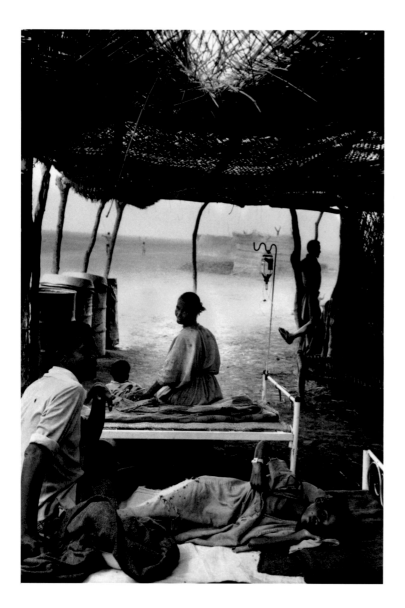

1985—(left) Fau 3 Refugee Camp Hospital, in the Sudan. A series of political, climatic, and medical calamities led to a disaster that claimed tens of thousands of victims. The practice encouraged by Western governments of growing cash crops ended in deforestation and soil erosion. Drought followed, and then famine. Relief food and medicine, withheld at first by the United States (reluctant to help a socialist regime), came late, or often failed to arrive. The local government commandeered supplies and used them as a political tool against the rebels. Delivering medical care outdoors is always a last resort. Photographed by David Heiden.

1949—(opposite) Wide-open spaces are frequently deemed to provide magical therapy, and the desert is reputed to work wonders. These were arthritis studies in Tucson, Arizona, where the dry climate is still thought to be beneficial to sufferers of a condition which continues to defy medicine's best efforts to locate either a cause or a cure. New studies point to the possibility that some forms of arthritis are probably autoimmune diseases, in which white blood cells mistakenly devour healthy cartilage in the joints. Photographed by Alfred Eisenstaedt.

sanitation, immunization, the early detection of disease, and increased community awareness is driven home by every overcrowded hospital and by every needless death.

But if modern medicine is tempted into a bit of smugness as it brings its own thinking to the developing countries, it is also taking away from them a humbling message. Western doctors have learned that in some spheres of illness, "primitive" people know secrets that have eluded medicine in the industrialized countries throughout all these years of progress. So the Westerners who have had the courage to head off into foreign lands, bearing gifts of their training, have brought back with them something to treasure, too, a new reverence for the human spirit as an agent of healing and a new belief that nature holds the key to medical therapies as yet unimagined.

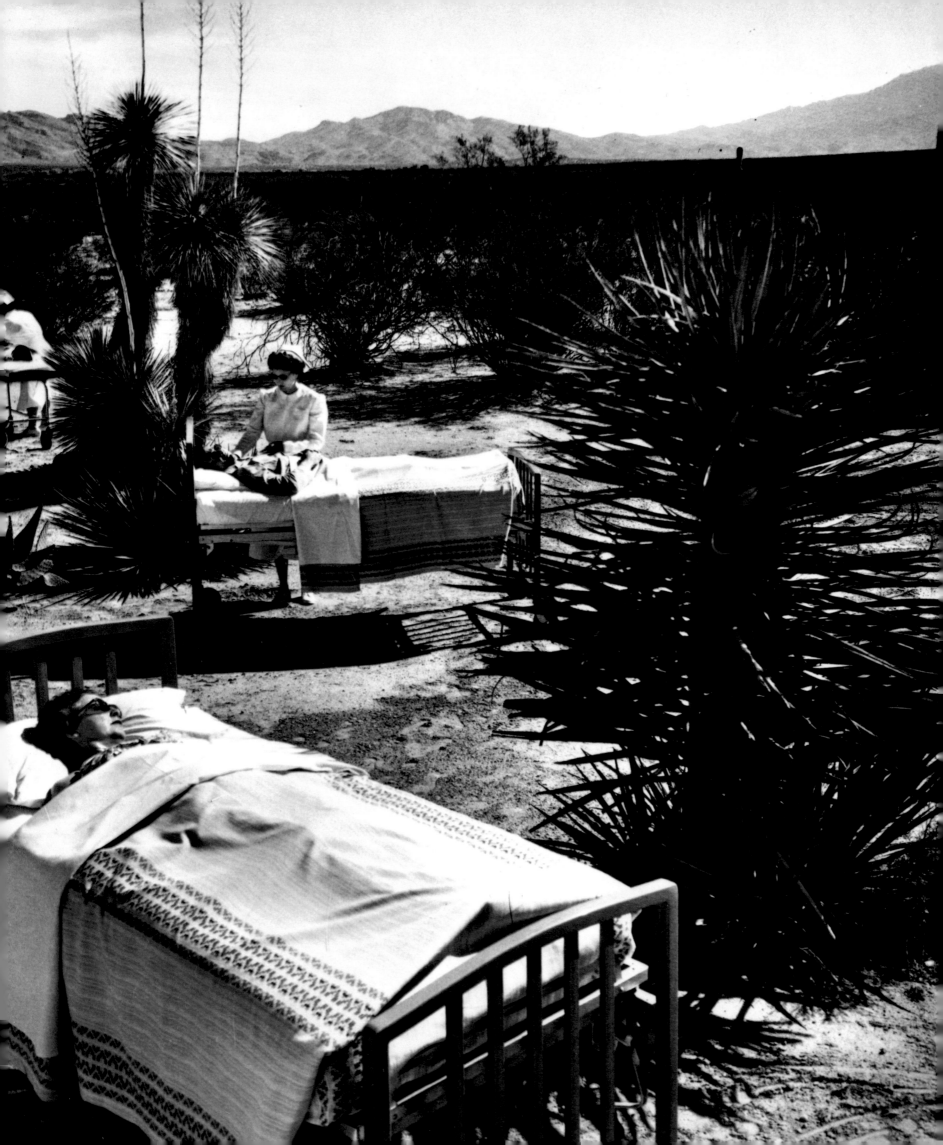

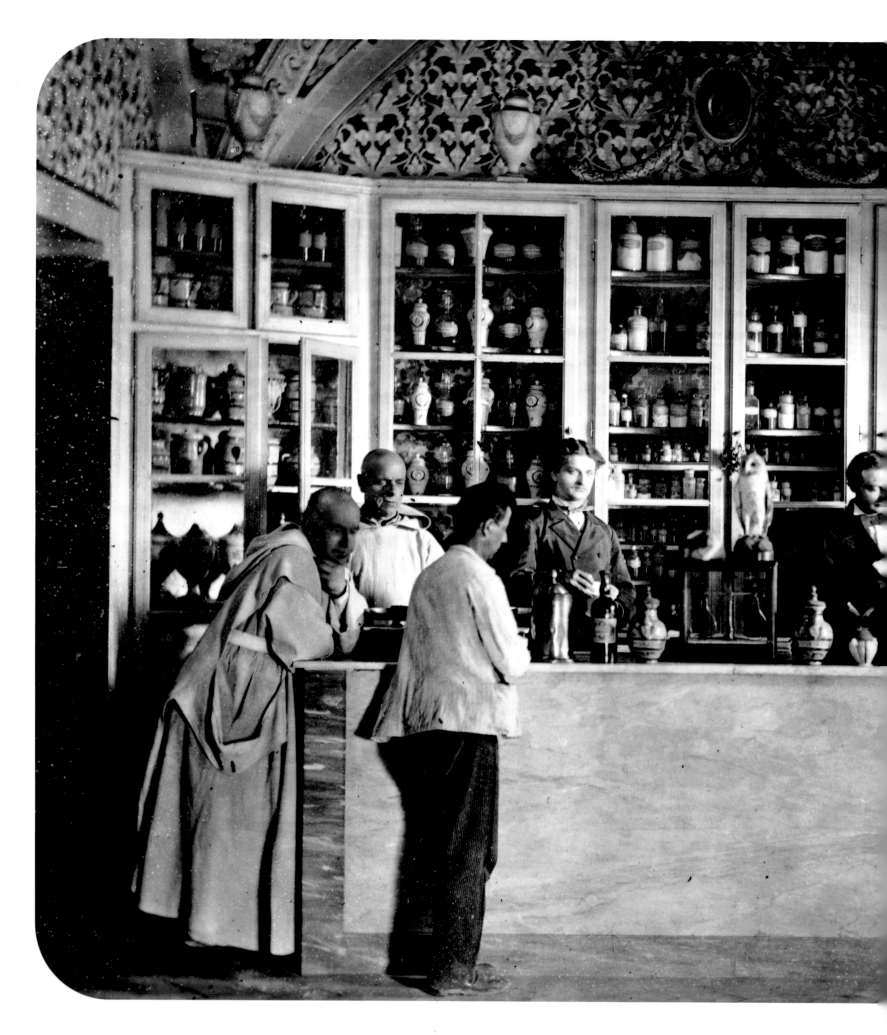

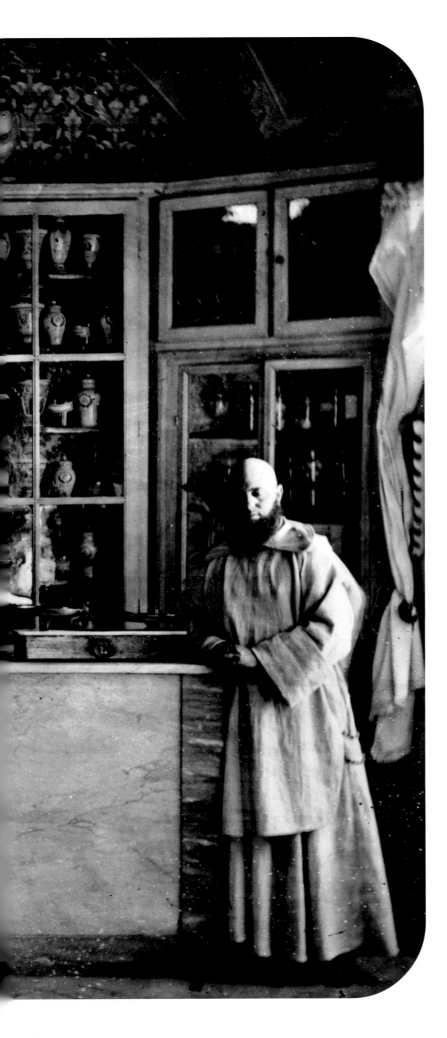

CHAPTER FOUR

THE TOOLS OF MEDICINE

FROM X RAYS TO MAGNETIC RESONANCE IMAGING, THE TOOLS OF MODERN MEDICINE HAVE EVOLVED TO TAKE THE GUESSWORK OUT OF DIAGNOSIS AND ENABLE TREATMENTS OF BREATHTAKING PRECISION. DRUGS, IN THE TWENTIETH CENTURY, FINALLY SHED THE SHROUD OF DARK-AGES QUACKERY AND PROVED THEY COULD DELIVER SO SPECTACULARLY THAT SOME OF THEM—WITH GOOD REASON—WOULD BE CALLED MIRACLE DRUGS.

The difference between today and a hundred years ago is even more startling in this area of drugs than it is with diagnostic tools. In the first and second decades of the century, a doctor's bag might have included only morphine for pain, digitalis to give the heart a boost, and perhaps insulin for diabetes. Quinine had been available to fight malaria since 1820, and a vaccine against smallpox had existed since 1798. A drug to fight diphtheria did not appear until 1890. Throughout this period, enemas, laxatives, and purgatives were heavily used by the physician although, despite a certain amount of discomfort that may have made them seem effective, they were largely useless.

While the ability to diagnose illness was increasing by great leaps, the drugs to effectively alleviate symptoms and cure and prevent disease were almost nonexistent in the first quarter of this century. Today, the doctor's bag is more metaphor than anything else. Pharmacies are routinely required to contain prescribed drugs of proven ability to fight everything from anxiety to pimples to pain. After World War I, the pharmaceutical industry grew into a global powerhouse, much of it centered in Europe.

Circa 1900—*In this pharmacy in Florence, Italy, as well as in others around the world, there were few truly effective drugs at the turn of the century. But the recent discovery and success of aspirin helped to fuel the pharmaceutical industry which soon began to produce other highly effective drugs.*

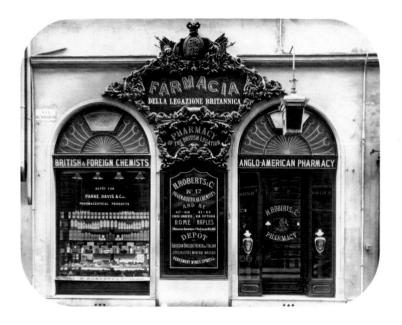

The mechanism for how some drugs work is well known, while other drugs are prescribed because they are demonstrably effective, even if the reasons for their efficacy reside more in the realm of hypothesis than in known fact. But it is a measure of how far medicine has come in providing drugs for human ills that many patients rebel against them because they seem too easy. "Take two aspirin and call me in the morning"—the standing joke about medical response—is a phrase grounded in a century's reality. Aspirin is truly a miracle drug if ever there was one.

In 1886 in Alsace (then Germany), an unidentified pharmacist at the Kalle Company, preparing a medicine for intestinal parasites, instead concocted something from a coal-tar derivative. The patient's stomach didn't improve much, but his fever declined. The German Bayer company soon latched onto this promising fever reducer and developed a variant, acetylsalicylic acid, which it called aspirin, a drug that helped fevers and was effective against headaches. Europe embraced the drug, and in 1903 Bayer took its aspirin-producing know-how to America, to a factory on New York's Hudson River. After World War I, Bayer's hegemony was split, with American aspirin going to Sterling Products and the German holdings to I.G. Farben. In 1920, when Judge *(continued on page 139)*

Circa 1900—*(above) Pharmacy of the British legation, Florence, Italy.*

Circa 1888—*(right) Analytical chemistry laboratory, School of Chemistry, University of Paris. Groundbreaking work was being done in the labs of France, but there, as elsewhere, cleanliness and sterility were the exceptions. Fastidiousness was slow in coming. Even in the 1920s, the esteemed Rockefeller University scientist Thomas Rivers felt compelled to complain about his working conditions, "as three women lab assistants have come down with psittacosis [parrot fever]."*

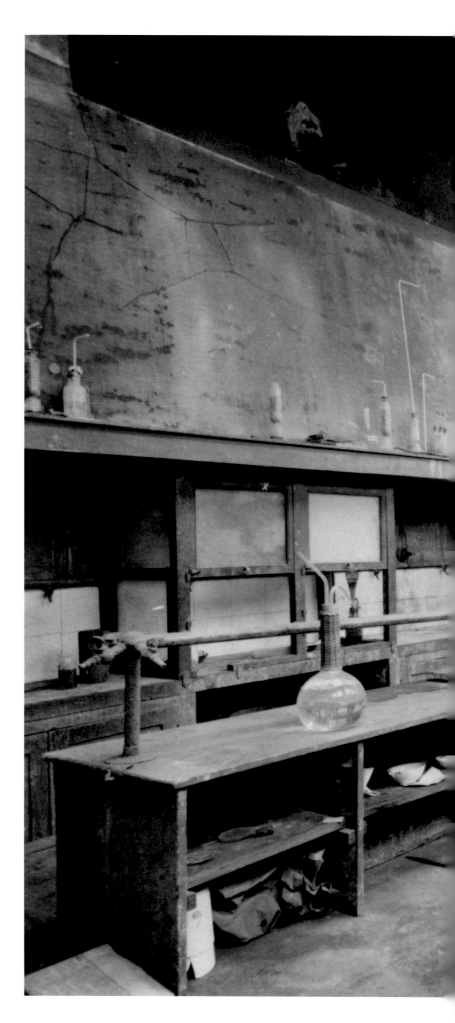

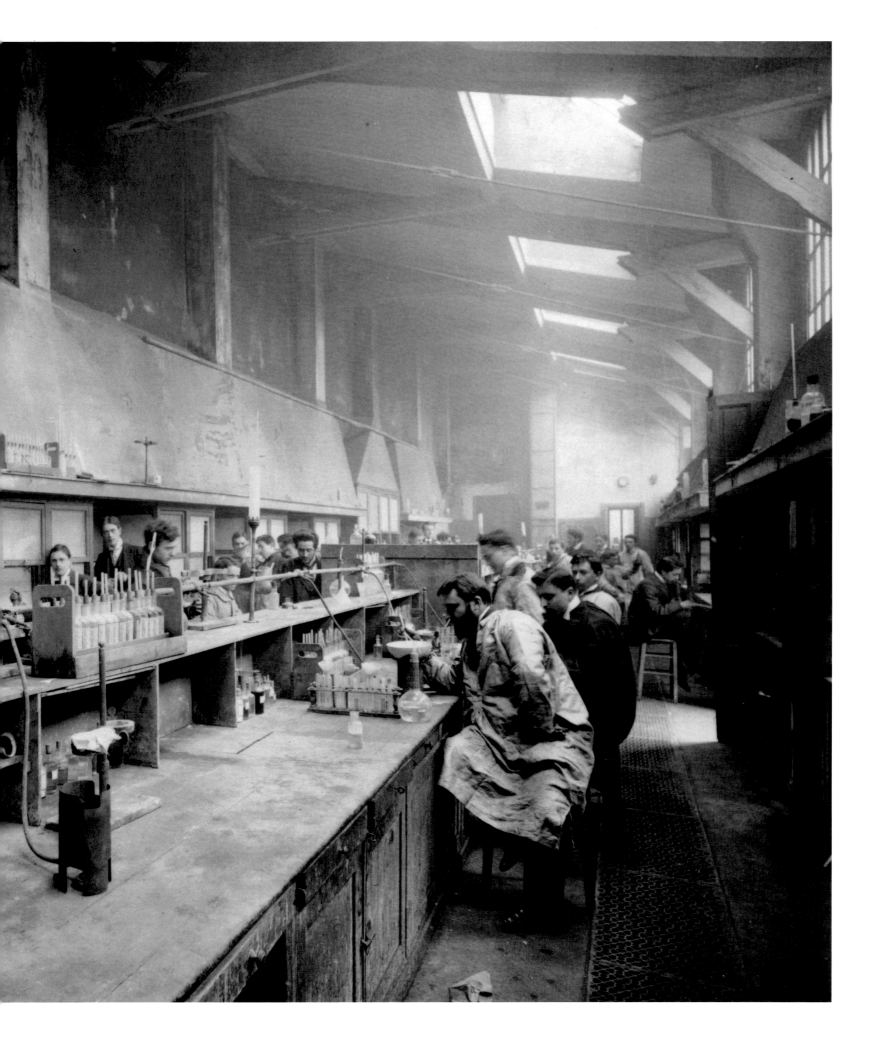

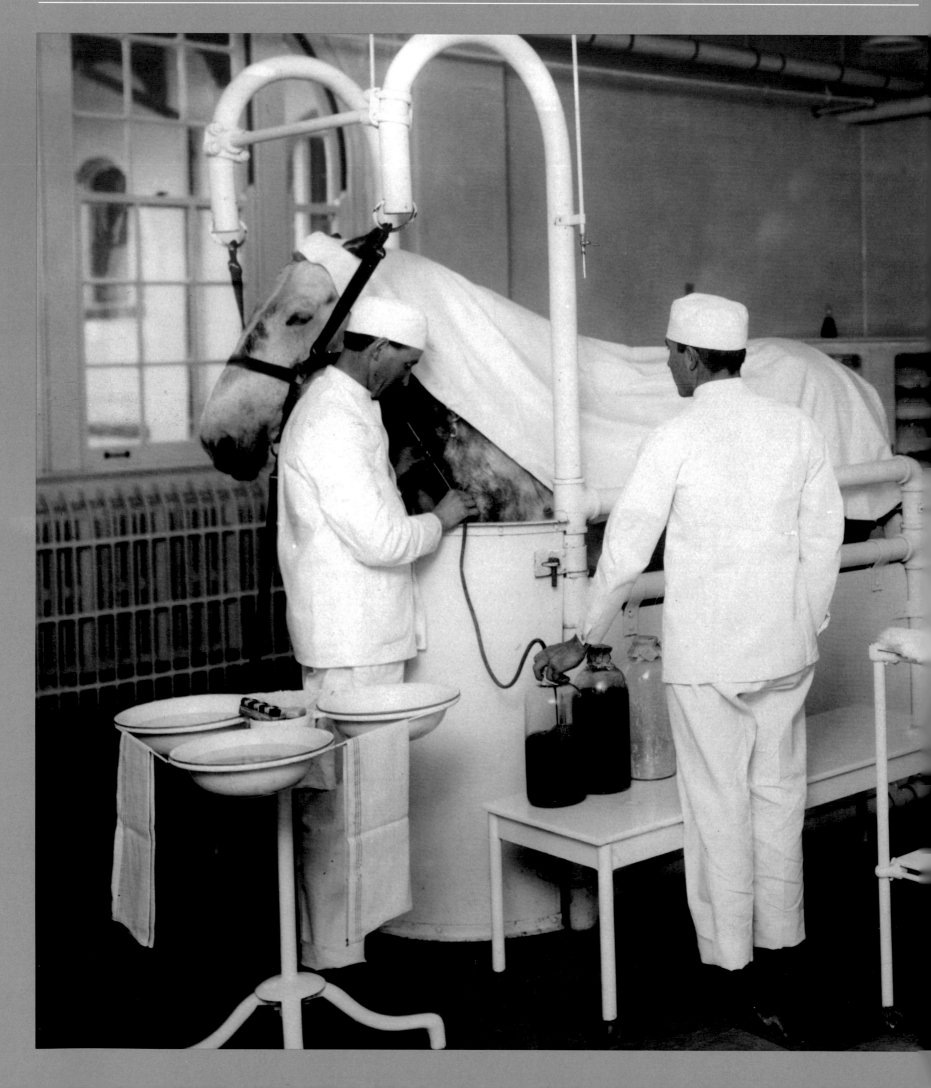

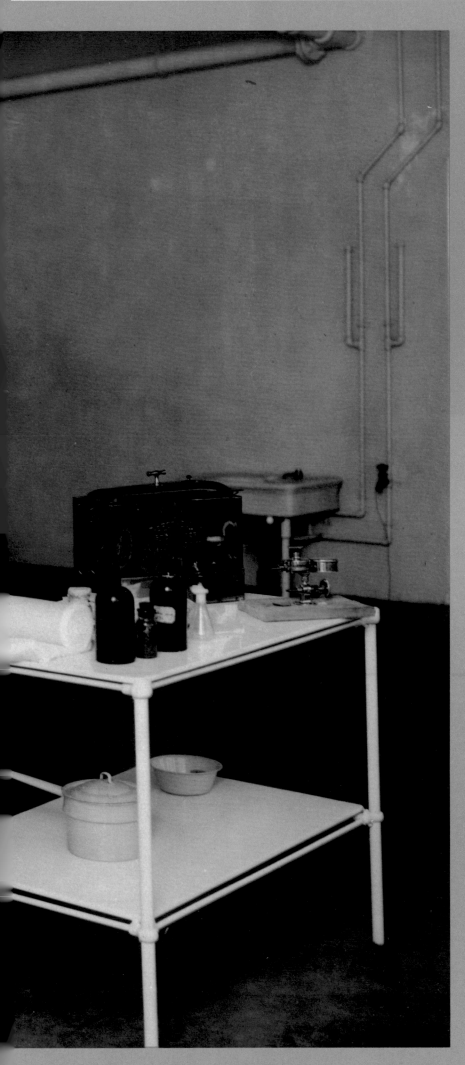

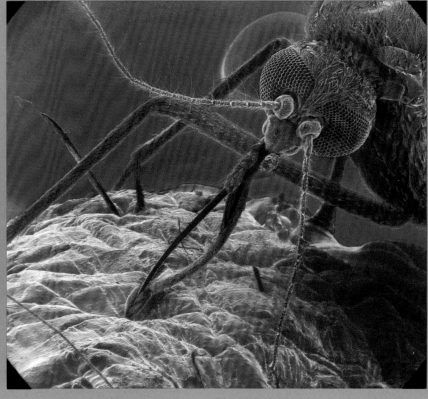

Blood Ties

1975—*(above)* Nature is bursting with the agents of infection and the vectors of disease. The Aedes mosquito, magnified forty-five times under the scanning electric microscope, is seen here caught in the act of extracting human blood and, perhaps, leaving a virus behind. Nature is increasingly being seen also as a source of salvation, a treasure trove of drugs—frequently extracted from plants in the wild—to fight illnesses of all kinds. Photographed by Lennart Nilsson.

1910—*(left)* It was nature, in the form of a mold inadvertently grown in the lab by an untidy bacteriologist named Alexander Fleming, that provided the world with penicillin. Animals too have often been the vehicle for producing important drugs. Here, in 1910, a horse donates blood so that scientists might obtain diphtheria antitoxin vaccine at a Lilly & Co. plant. The animal was first induced to develop antibodies that could be employed to activate the human immune system.

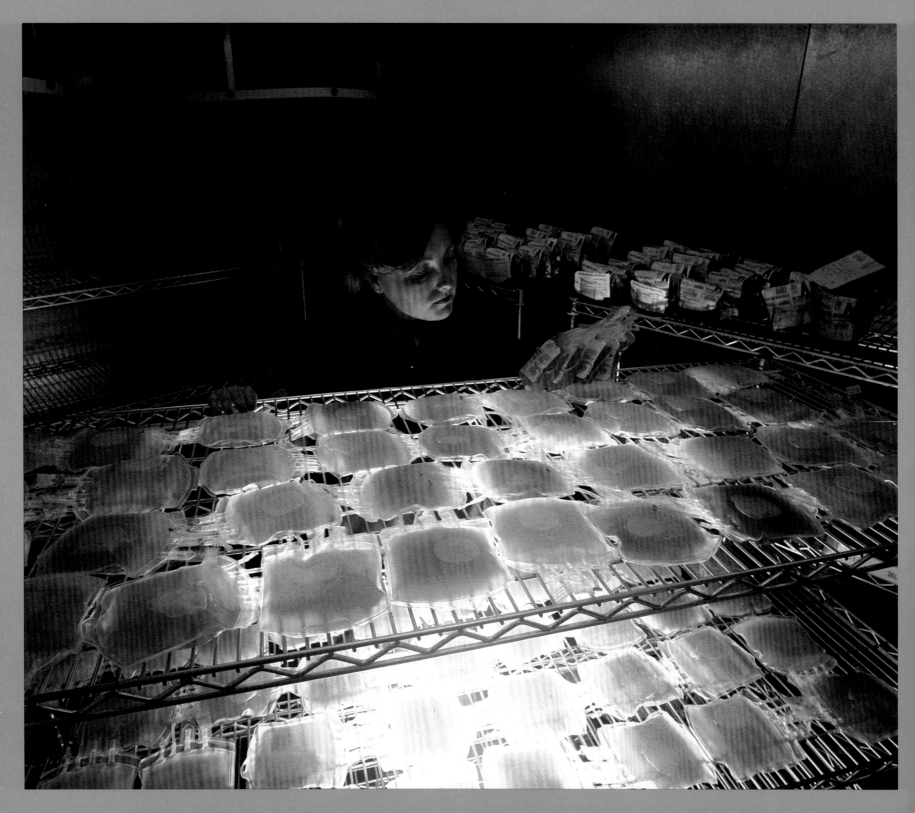

1989—*(above)* Although one usually doesn't think of it that way, nature is at work when human beings donate blood to each other. Donated human blood has become a linchpin of surgery and is also central to the treatment of some diseases. In fact, without the development of blood transfusion, no major surgery would be possible at all. The processing of blood has become increasingly sophisticated, involving techniques for removing components of whole blood that were developed during World War II. In some cases, the clotting component alone, factor VIII, is removed from whole blood and administered to hemophiliacs. Through efficient use and storage of such blood components, thousands of lives are saved each year. Photographed by Nathan Benn.

1984—*(opposite)* Of all the tools that have transformed modern medicine, the helicopter's influence in medical trauma care is among the most dramatic: fast, agile, and roaring. This American Red Cross helicopter can rush blood and medical equipment to a distant emergency. And in this instance, it rushed two critically injured people to a hospital 520 miles away. Photographed by Annie Griffiths Belt.

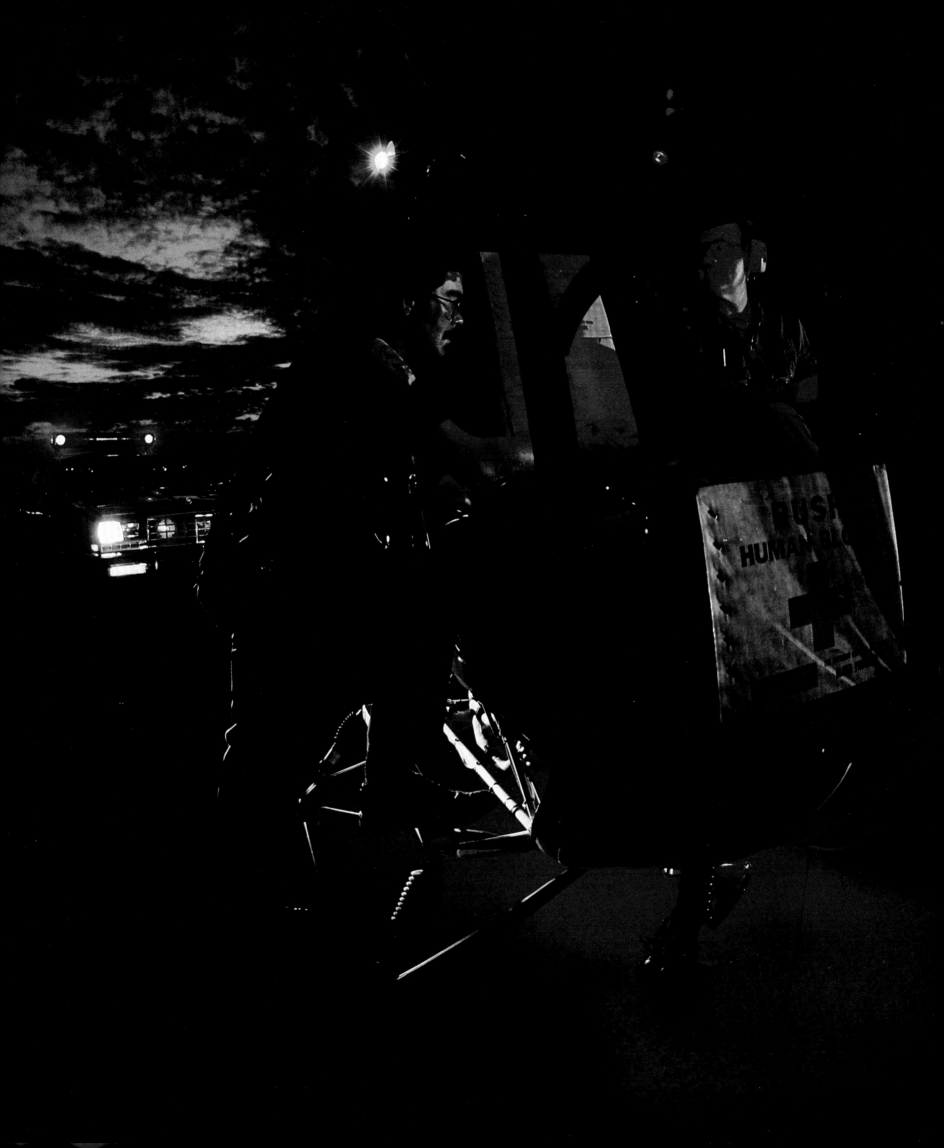

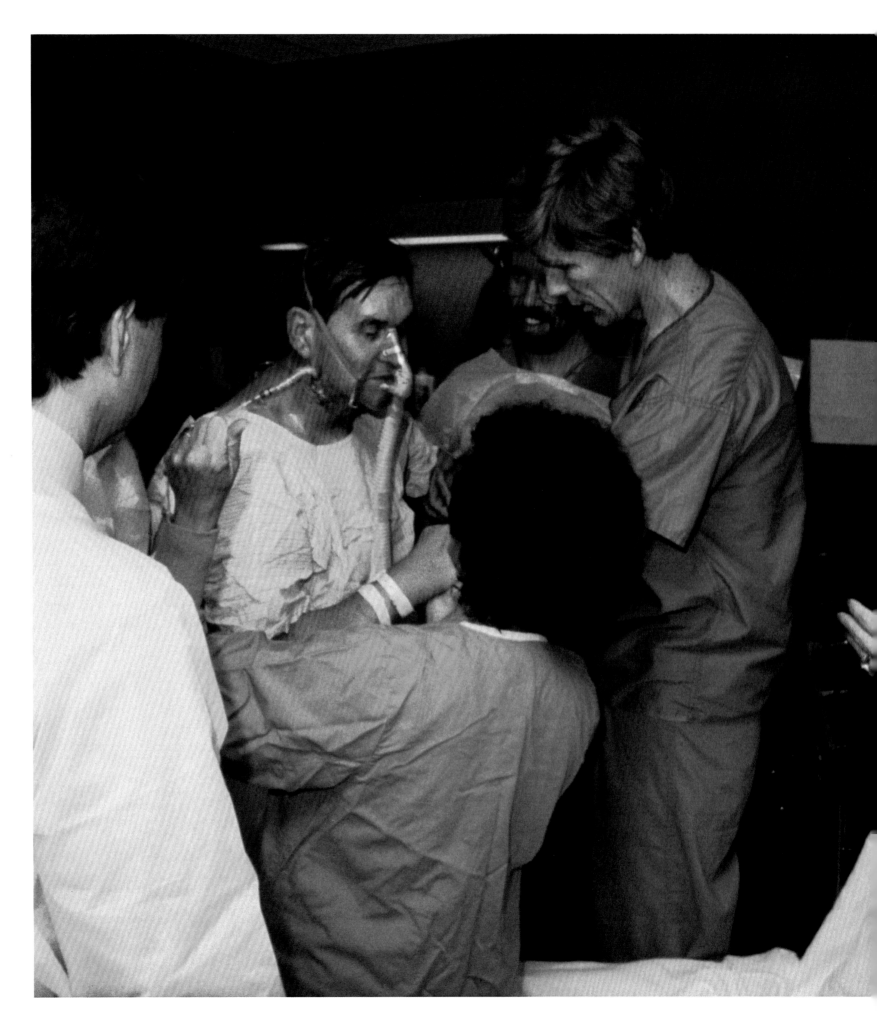

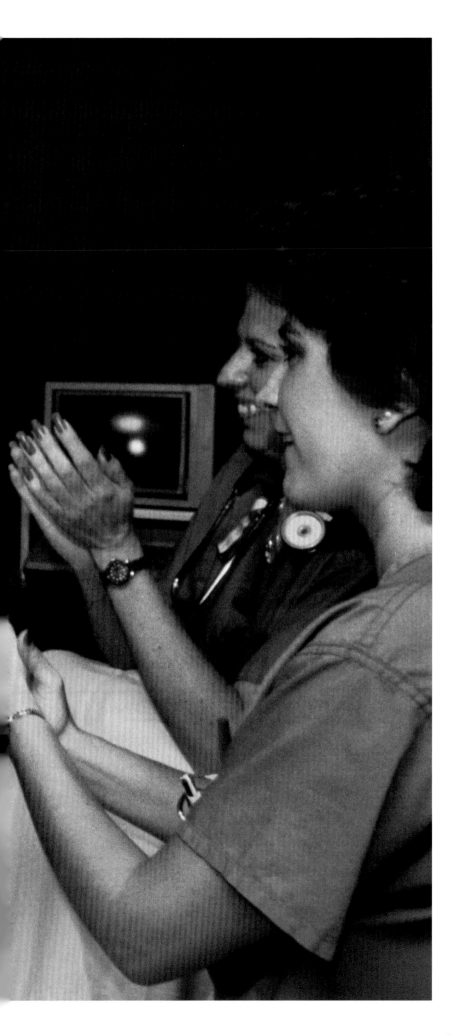

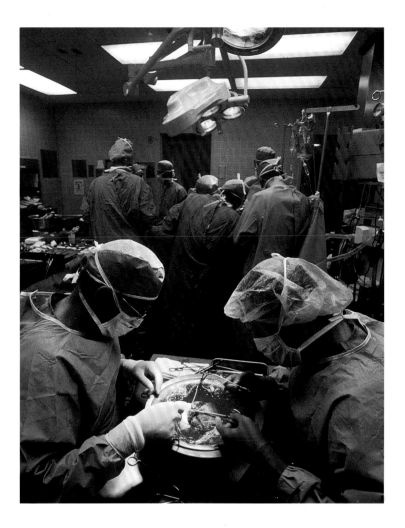

Learned Hand ruled that the public treated "aspirin" as if it was a generic name, the word itself was permitted to be used by any company. Along with vitamins, this wonder drug sparked a significant expansion in the pharmaceutical industry.

And a strange drug it turned out to be, lowering the temperature of sick people but not those who are well. Time would reveal that aspirin possessed other properties, too. In 1950, Dr. Lawrence I. Craven, a California physician, noticed an unusual amount of bleeding in some of his tonsillectomy patients. He attributed it to the aspirin in Aspergum (chewable aspirin) and

---

1984—(left) An astonishing machine that almost worked: the artificial heart. The patient, William Schroeder, takes his first step following the insertion of a mechanical heart, powered from outside the body. He is assisted by Dr. William De Vries, the leading proponent of the technique. The death of all of Dr. De Vries's patients marked a disappointing chapter in recent medical history. Photographed by William Strode.

1992—(above) While the hopes for artificial hearts were dashed, liver transplants became one of the century's true miracles. Here, at the University of Chicago Medical Center, Rick Goykin has donated a piece of his liver to replace the diseased organ of his nineteen-month-old daughter, Nicole. Photographed by Bill Luster.

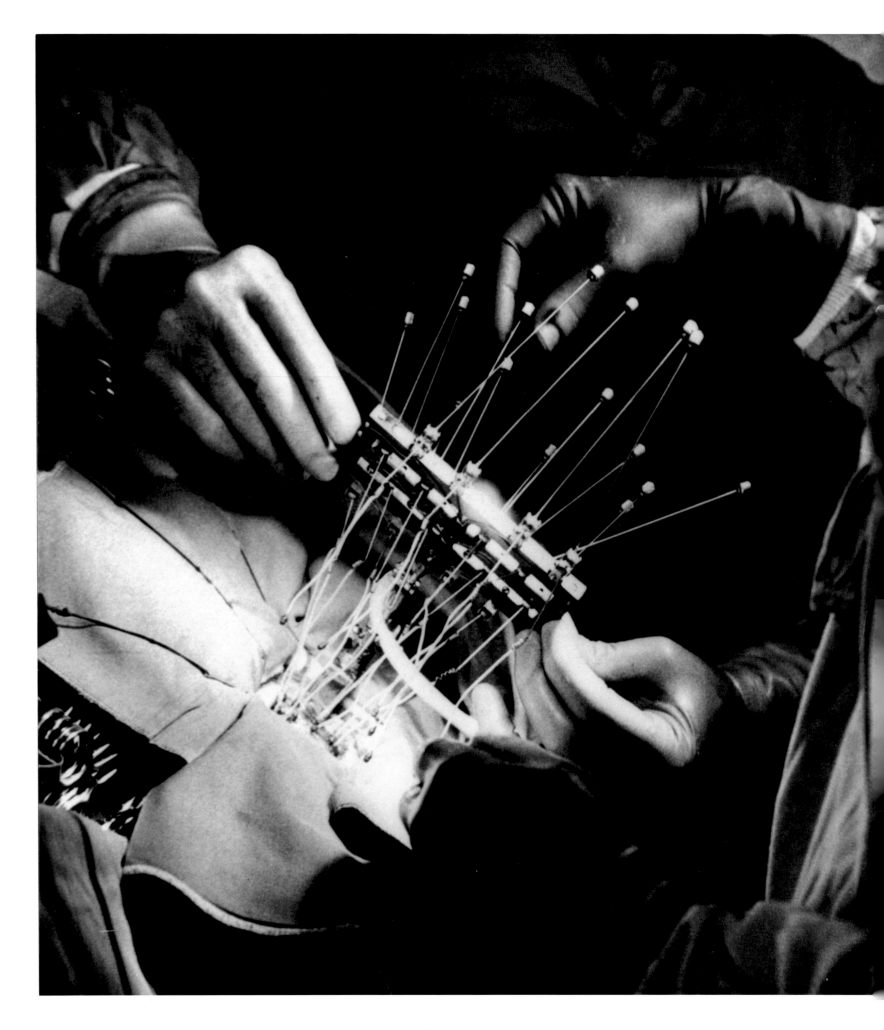

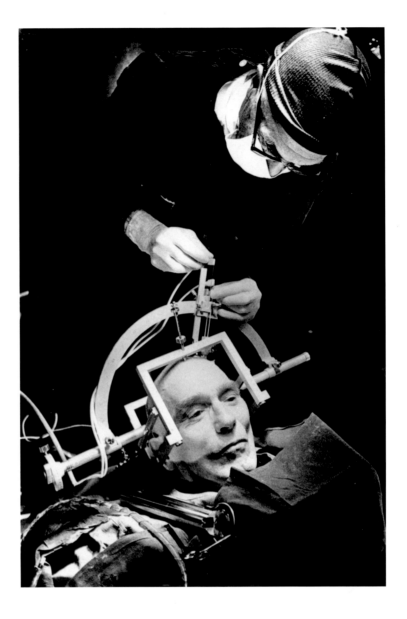

1963—*(left) The still incompletely understood brain remains a frontier of modern medicine. At the behavioral level, ideas and thoughts originate in the cortex and are expressed in language and gesture. At the microscopic level, the brain's 200 billion nerve cells are activated in intricate patterns that one scientist whimsically called "an enchanted loom." On a molecular level, the brain's chemical messengers, around sixty neurotransmitters, stimulate, inhibit, or change communication. These three levels are still a mystery though we have learned more in the last fifty years than in the previous 500. Here, electrodes record the brain's activity during surgery. Photographed by Fred Ward.*

1965—*(above) Life-devastating Parkinson's disease— causing problems with balance, muscle control, and speech—has preoccupied many brain scientists around the world, preeminent among them the surgeons at Karolinska Sjukhuset, Stockholm, Sweden, who are preparing a patient for surgery. Photographed by Lennart Nilsson.*

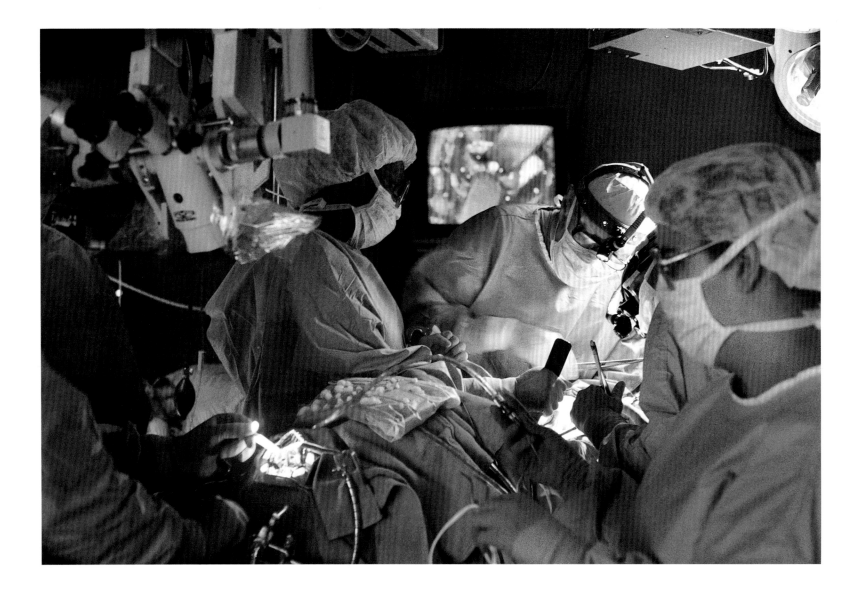

figured that if aspirin was responsible for reduced clotting, it might work in preventing heart attacks. But that insight awaited research in the eighties to demonstrate that a bit of aspirin every other day does seem to prevent heart attacks and, moreover, is linked to diminished risk of colon cancer.

Drug development throughout the world, like medical research, has not taken a straight line from triumph to triumph. Instead, there have been frequent failures in which side effects proved disastrous and promised benefits proved illusory. At the same time, the preponderance of the evidence has pointed toward improvements in health dramatic enough to radically alter the way a particular ailment, symptom, or class of diseases is viewed. Many drugs have emerged in the past century, whose influence on our lives can be underlined by noting the effects of just a few.

The arrival at mid-century of extraordinarily effective mind drugs, like Halperidol, known commercially as Haldol, that quiet the demons of schizophrenia led to the release of mental patients from institutions and often, lamentably, into a wasted life on the streets when they failed to maintain the *(continued on page 157)*

1989—*(above) After groundbreaking work on Parkinson's disease by surgeons in Mexico, doctors at Vanderbilt University Medical Center in Nashville, Tennessee, offered experimental surgery to a few patients. Two operations on Allen Northington proceed simultaneously. The first is the removal of adrenal tissue, which produces the brain chemical called dopamine, and the second is the transplantation of that tissue into the patient's brain. Photographed by Lynn Johnson.*

1984—*(opposite) Another surprising procedure at the frontier of medicine: radial keratotomy, a laser operation to cure near-sightedness. It was developed in the Soviet Union, took hold tentatively in the United States, and gradually has become a more established procedure worldwide. Photographed by Charles O'Rear.*

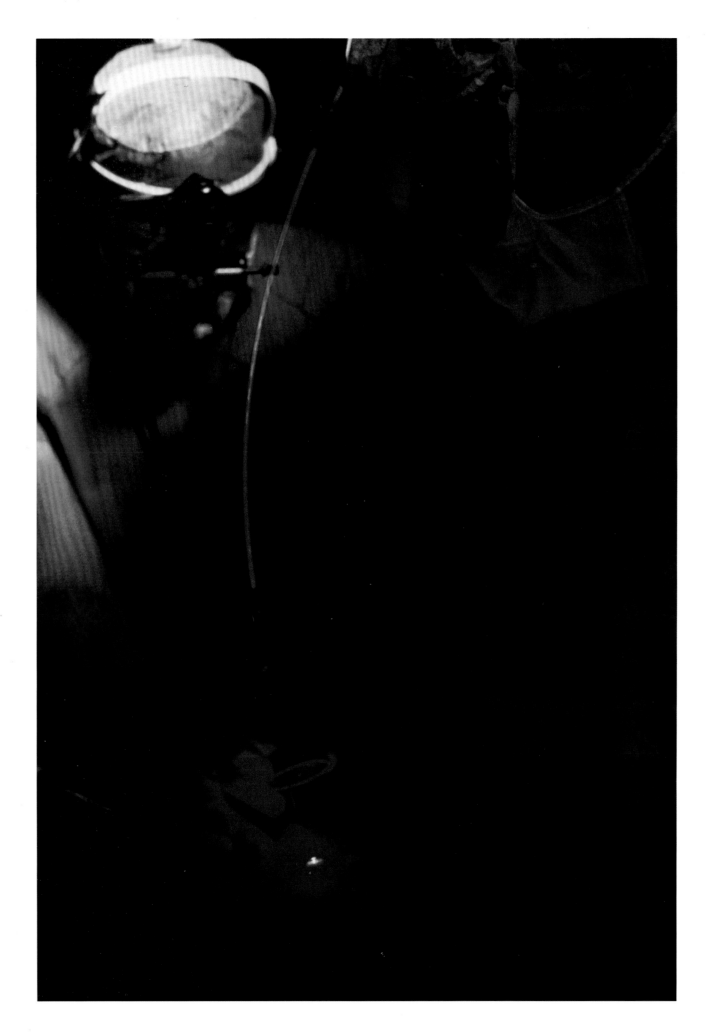

Pulleys, Cranks, and Ray Guns: A Portfolio of Incredible Machines

Doctors have always been assisted by machines—gadgets from the most pedestrian to the most farfetched, from the minimally useful to the startlingly efficient. As often as not, the match-up between people and machines is strange looking, indeed.

1936—*(below)* Monitoring the health of infants involves regular weighing. A nurse at Rose Bay Baby Health Center in Sydney, Australia balances the scale.

1988—*(right)* Modern day babies are subjected to a battery of tests. Here, a baby is settled onto three hundred gallons of warm water that will facilitate the obtaining of ultrasound images of his kidneys and spine. Eight sound emitters at the tank's bottom scan the body in regular slices. The device can detect abnormalities from tumors to cysts and hernias, as well as defects of the heart and kidneys. Photographed by Alexander Tsiaras.

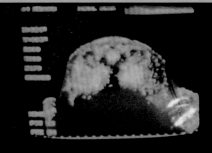

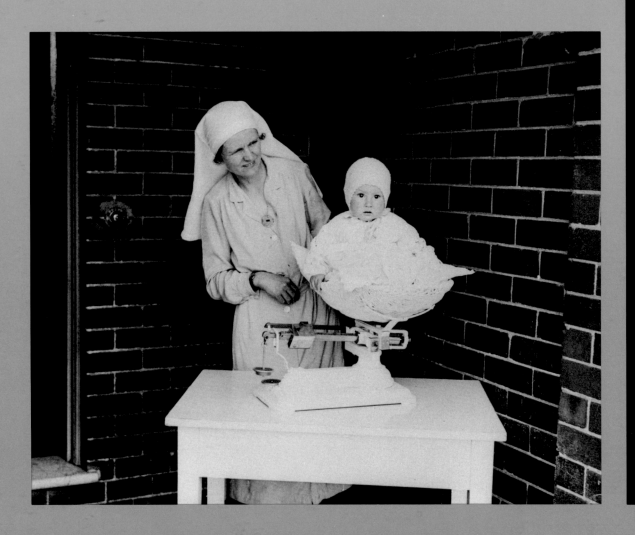

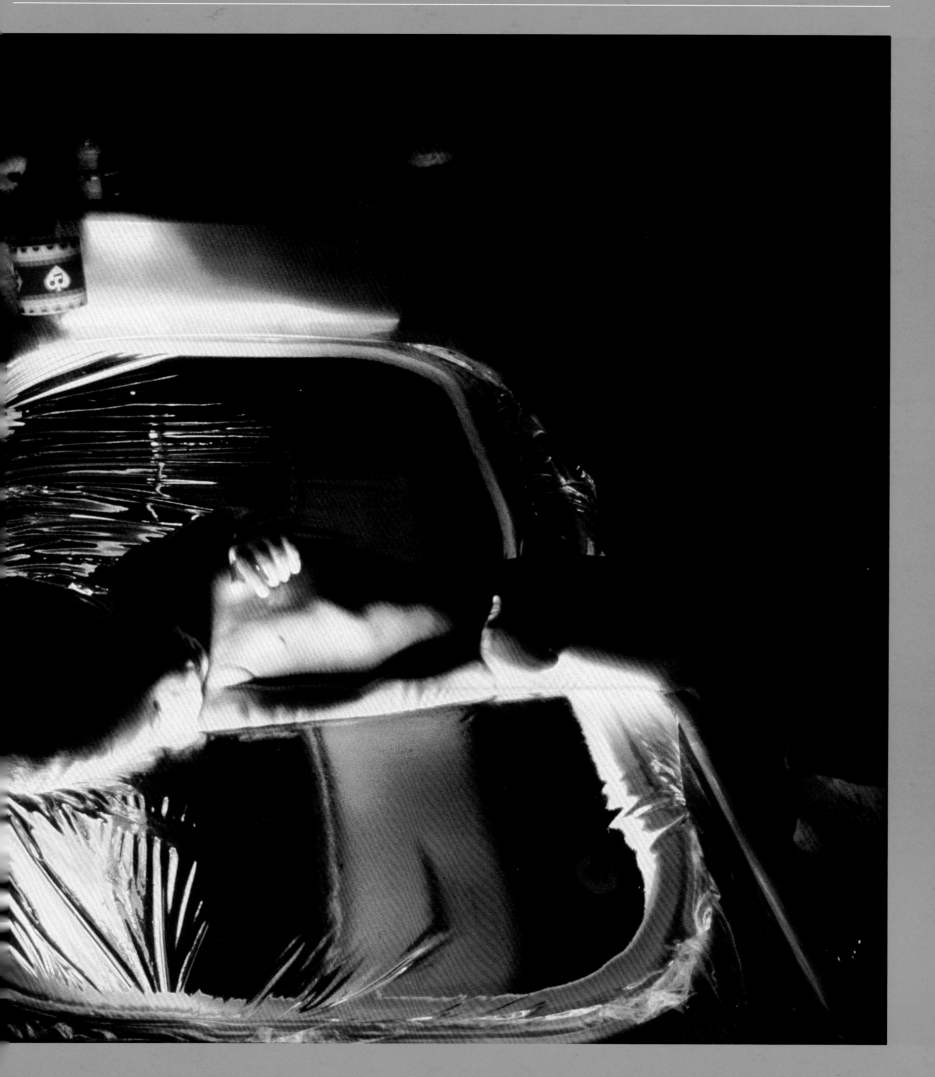

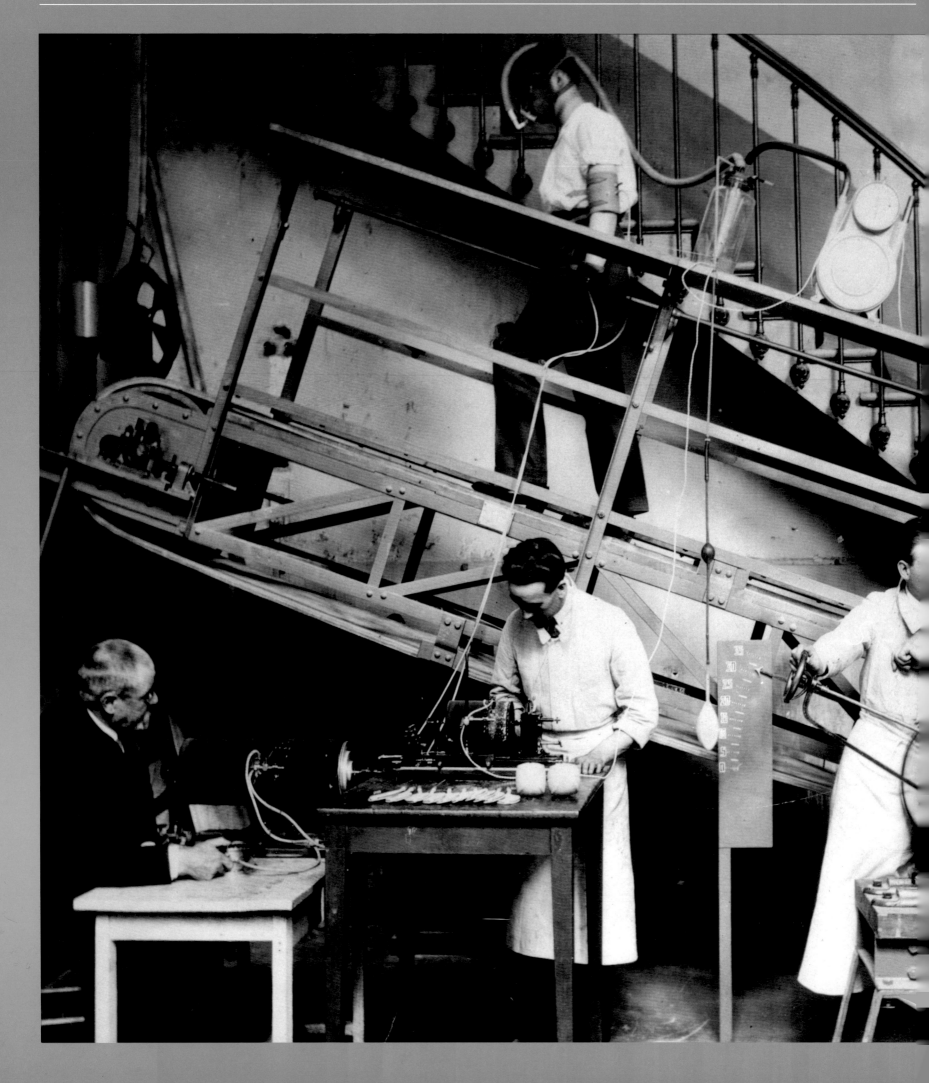

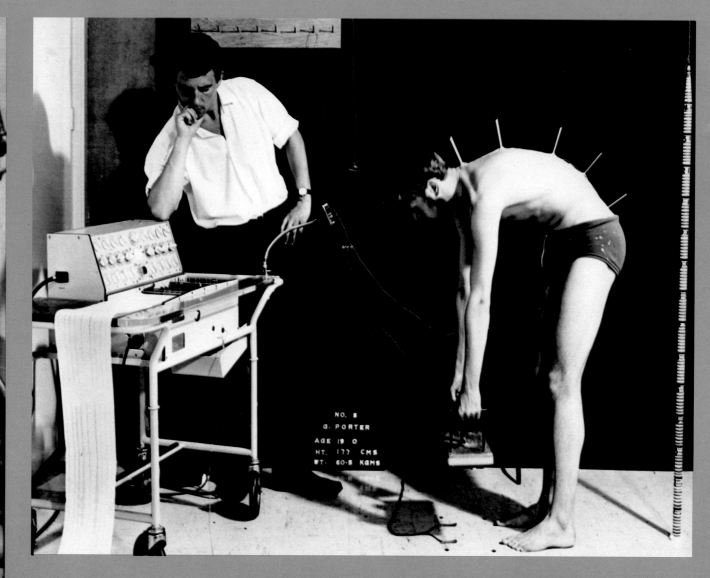

NO. 8
G. PORTER
AGE 19 0
HT. 177 CMS
WT. 60·5 KGMS

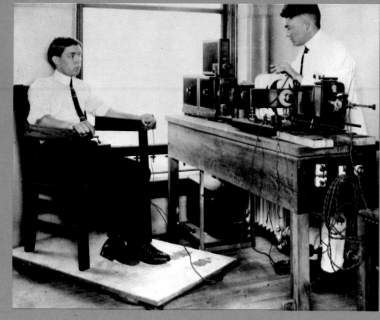

Circa 1930—*(far left)* Turning to what seems to be an early version of the modern stress test, a researcher in Paris runs an experiment in which a man pushes a wheelbarrow up an incline. He wears a mask that carries the expired air into an analysis jar; meanwhile, his pulse and blood pressure are monitored.

Circa 1959—*(above)* The vexatious human back is analyzed in a load-lifting test devised by British scientists.

1913—*(left)* The first electrocardiogram is performed in Chicago at Presbyterian Hospital.

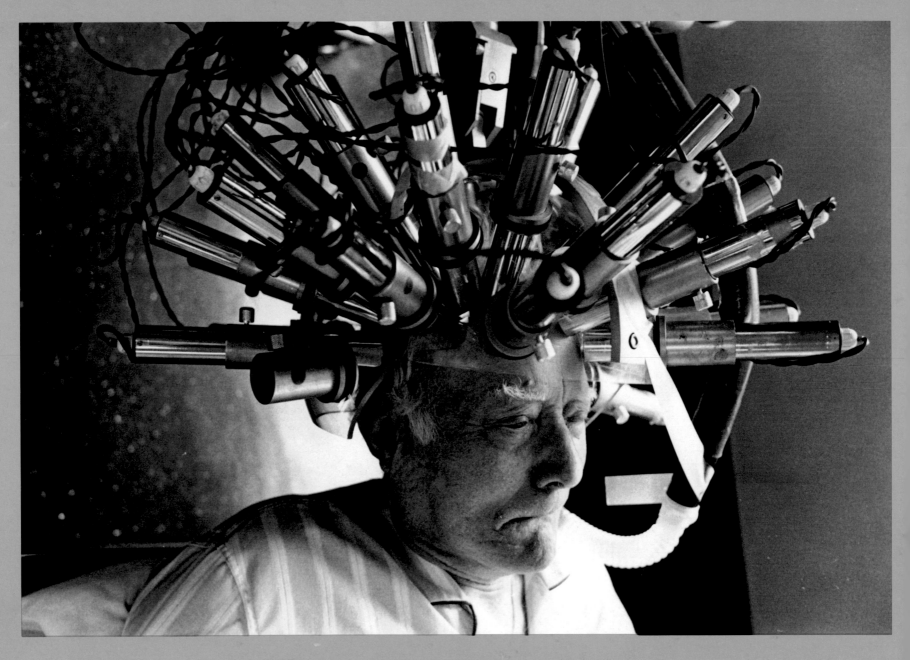

Circa 1960—*(above)* One of the wildest-looking contraptions in use today is seen here as it is employed in Toulouse, France, to measure blood circulation.

Circa 1930—*(opposite)* A test with a swinging ball in which a doctor seems to be either examining his patient's reflex reactions or hoping for a hypnotic trance. Photographed by Gordon Coster.

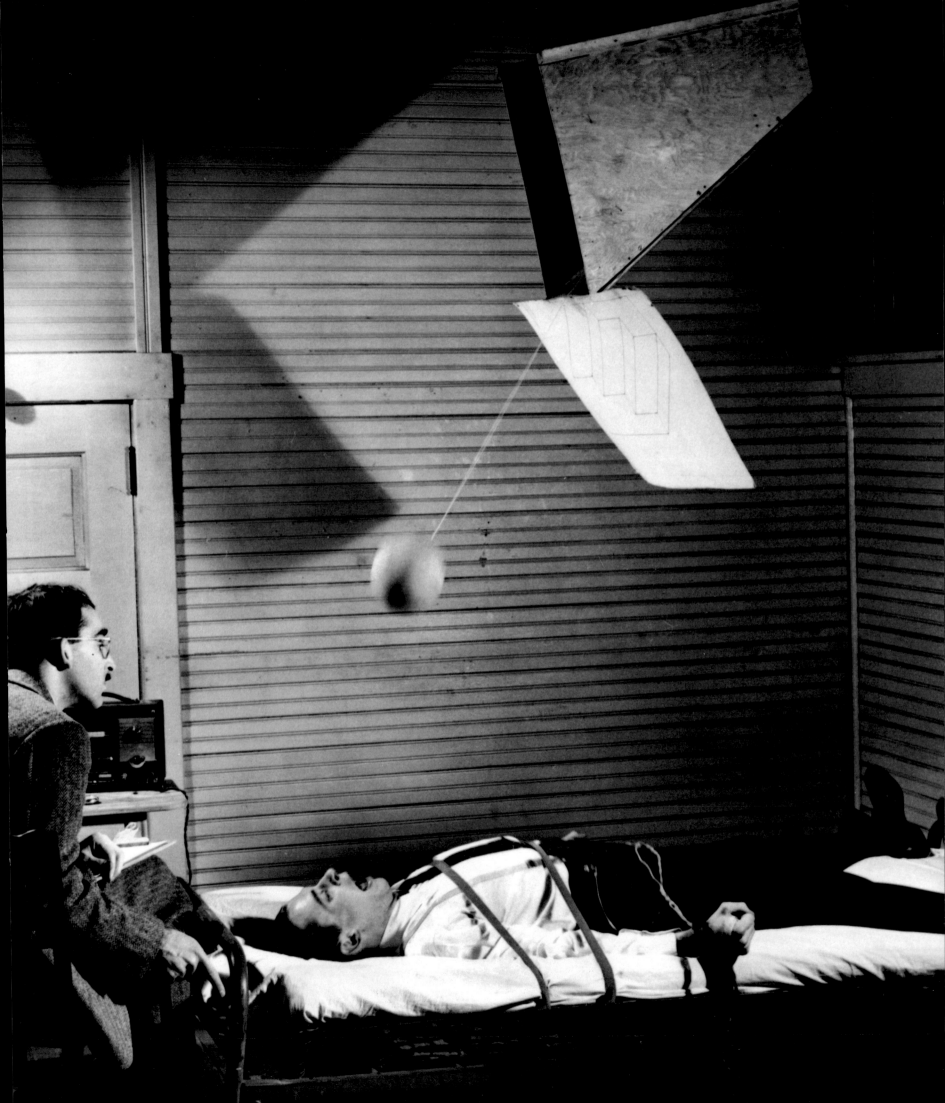

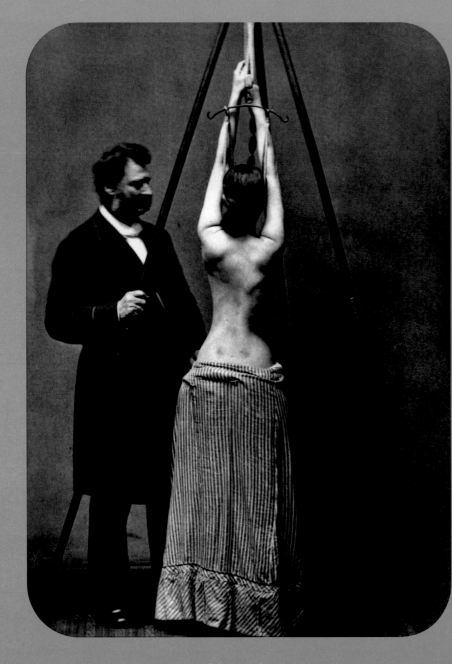

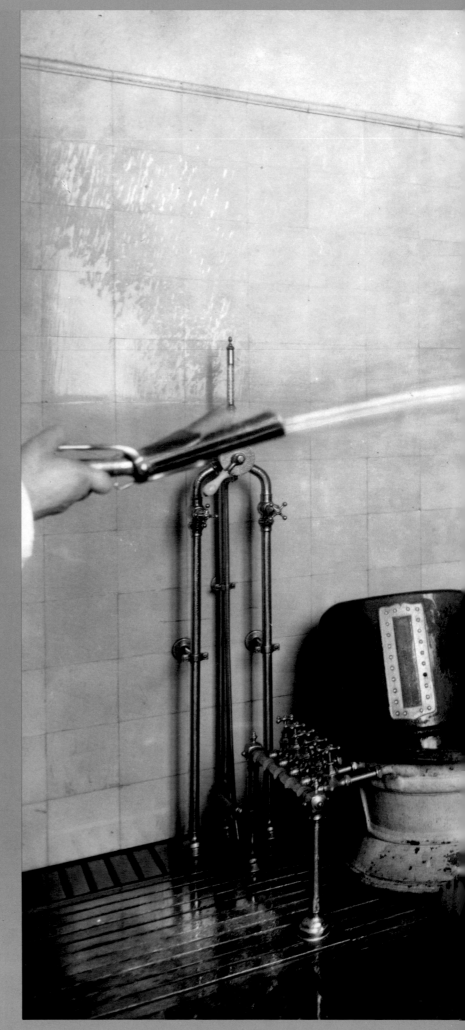

1877—*(above)* Scoliosis, a curvature of the spine that occurs at birth, was attended to by the esteemed Dr. Lewis Sayre, one of the fathers of American orthopedics. The patient is being prepared for a plaster cast in a demonstration of treatment at London's Royal Orthopedic Hospital. Photographed by J. P. Mayall.

1900—*(right)* At the baths of Montecatini, Italy, the backside of a patient is sprayed by a powerful hose. Water therapy was immensely popular as a cure for whatever ailed people, though it probably didn't cure anything.

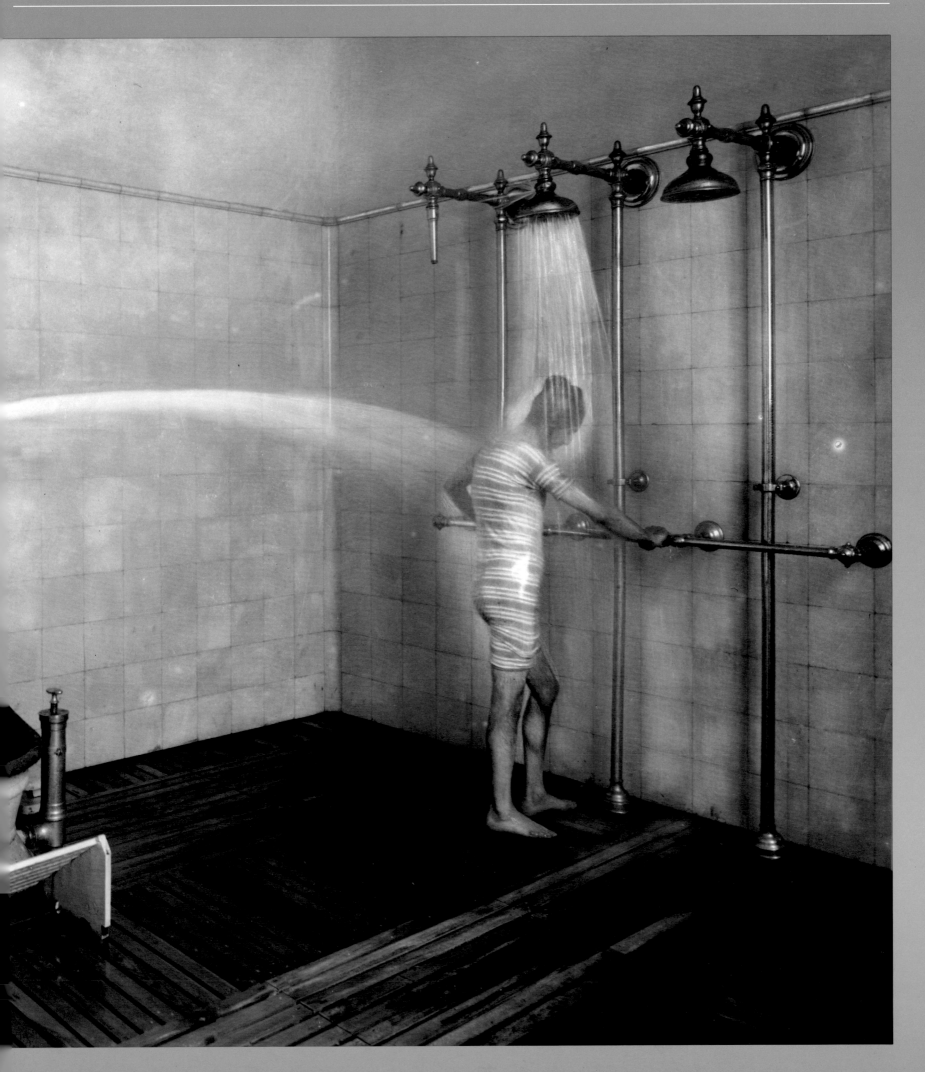

Circa 1910—*(below)* A primitive oxygen tent, shown here as it assisted a child at Toronto's Hospital for Sick Children. This was the precursor of a truly valuable tool, a staple of every modern medical care facility.

Circa 1930—*(right)* Mannequin with a light therapy lamp.

1910—*(far right)* The Foundling Hospital for Mothers and Infants in Milan, Italy. Light therapy, called "heliotherapy" earlier in the century, was another supposedly helpful approach to a number of ailments, and it did turn out to have some uses. Ultraviolet radiation was a means of treating rickets and dermatological problems and today is especially valuable to treat jaundice in infants.

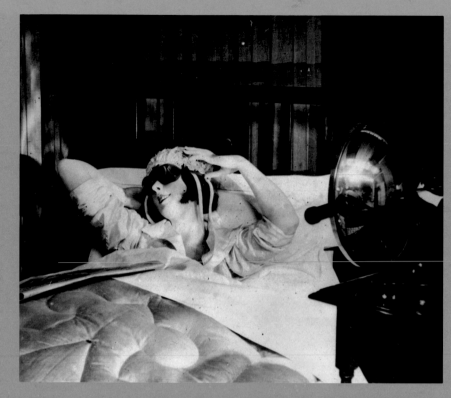

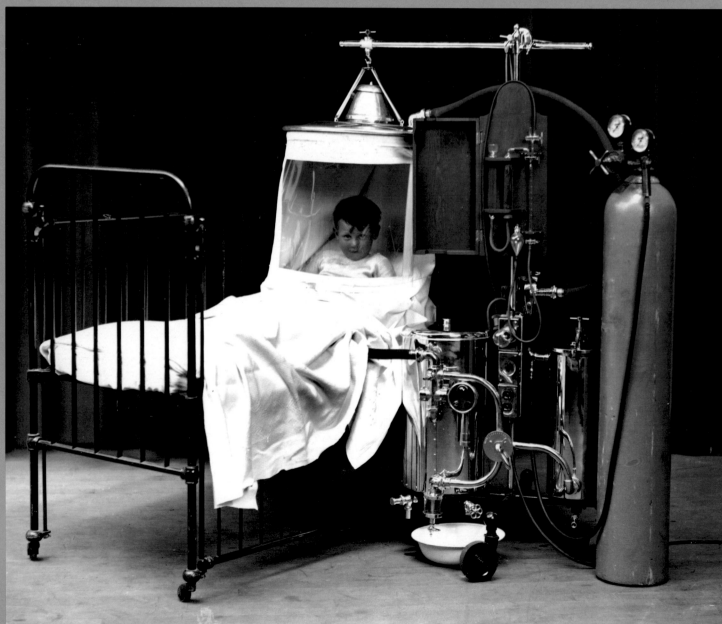

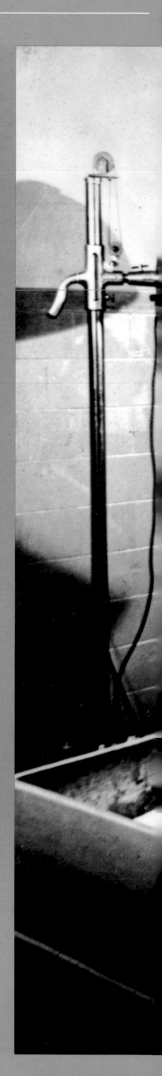

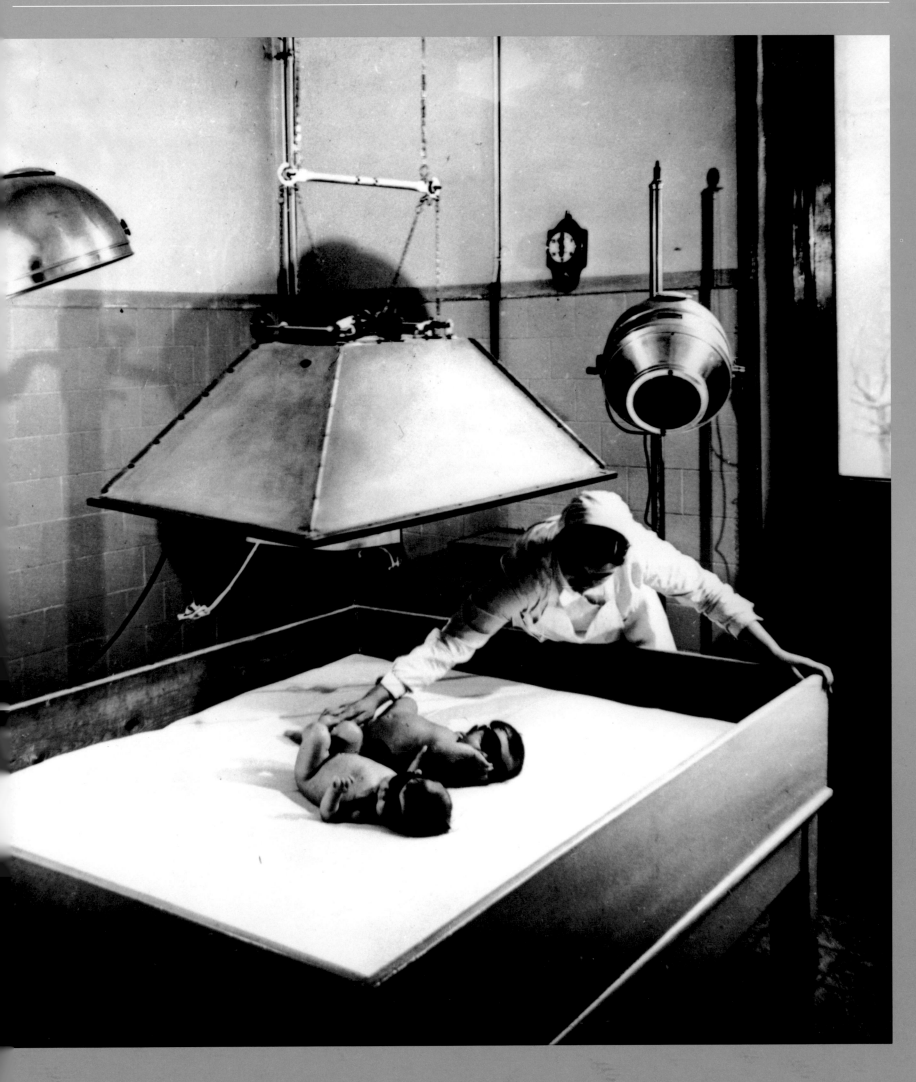

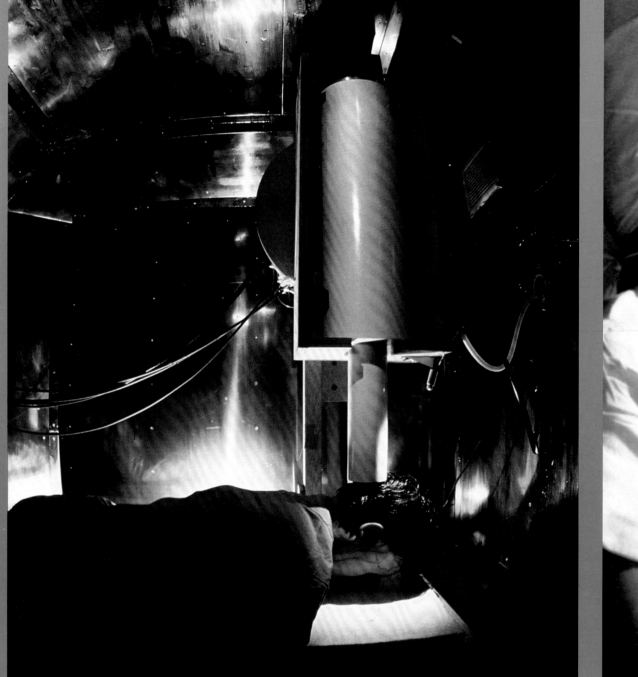

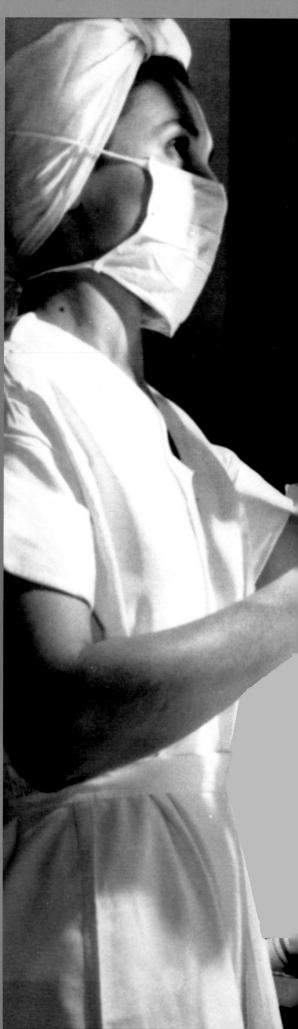

1989—*(above)* Expanding the frontiers of medicine in Japan, a powerful magnetometer called a SQUID uses superconductors to locate neural activity by detecting extremely weak magnetic fields in the brain. Photographed by Charles O'Rear.

Circa 1944—*(right)* This device that looks like a monstrous nutmeg grater is actually a magnet that a nurse in the operating room of a Minneapolis hospital is using to remove pieces of steel from a patient's eye.

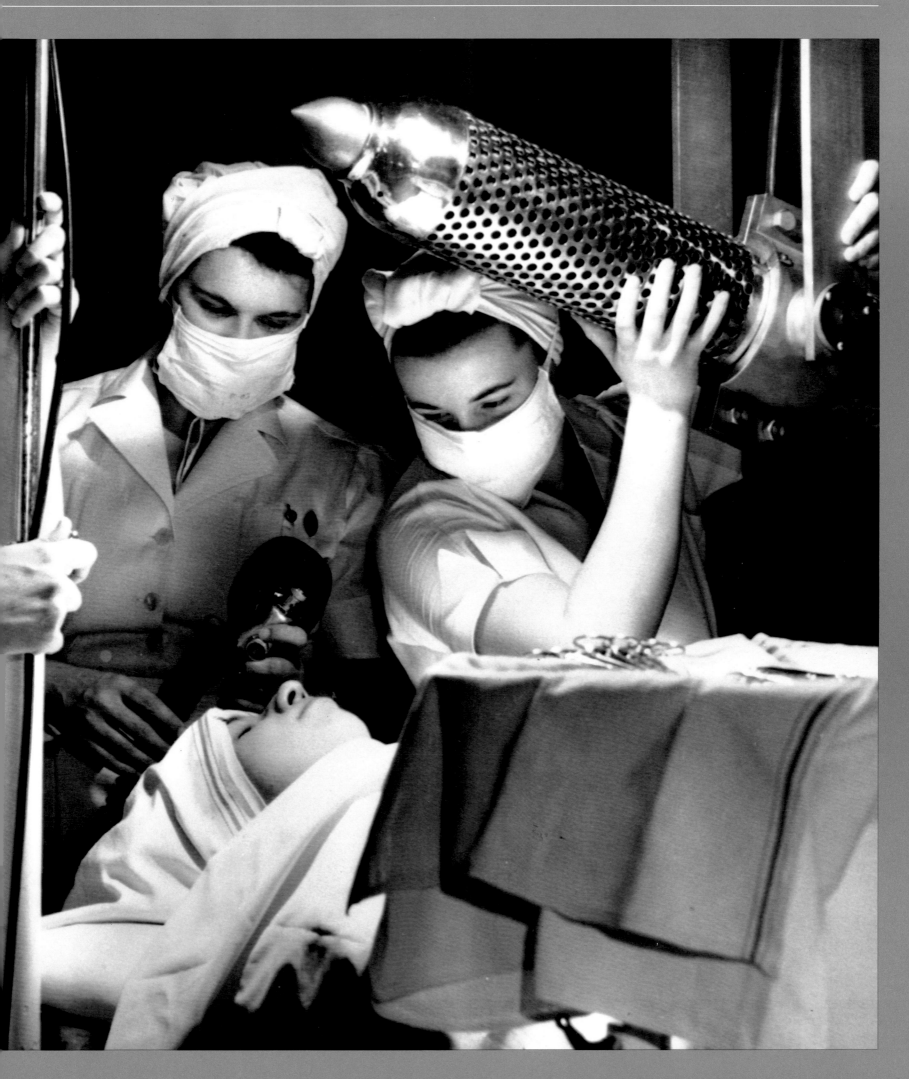

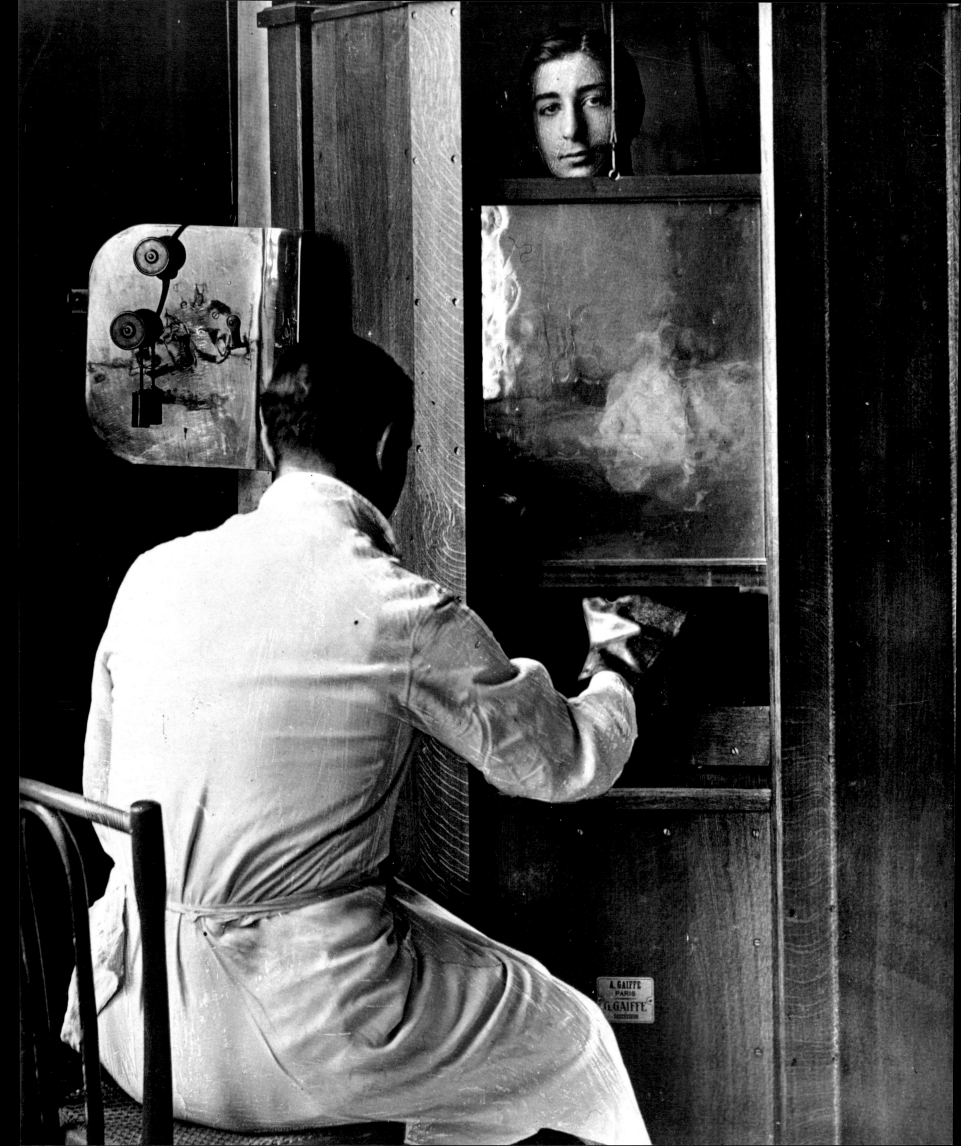

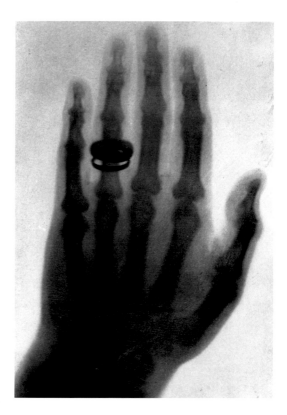

1914—*(opposite) An early X-ray apparatus at Cochin Hospital in Paris protects both the face and the rib cage of the young patient in a cabinet.*

Circa 1895—*(above) Wilhelm Konrad Roentgen, then professor of physics at the University of Würzburg, discovered the X ray in 1895. A staple in most of the progressive hospitals worldwide by the early twentieth century, Roentgen's discovery grandfathered the science of biomedical engineering, which expanded to include machines for ultrasound, tomography, and dialysis. Here, the first, famous, experimental X-ray image of Madame Roentgen's hand, complete with wedding ring. Photographed by Wilhelm Konrad Roentgen.*

drug regimen. Minor tranquilizers in the benzodiazepine family—Valium, Xanax, Halcion—were the most effective drugs ever devised against such problems as anxiety, panic disorder, and stage fright, but they proved to be far more addictive than researchers had at first believed.

Oral contraceptives blocked pregnancy, calcium channel blockers diminished the pain of angina, cortisone quieted inflammation, cyclosporine facilitated organ transplants, antihistamines made allergies bearable. But for unvarnished power in revolutionizing medicine, nothing could compare to the development of antibacterial agents. Until they came along, medicine, more often than not, could diagnose and alleviate, but could not cure. In 1927, Gerhard Domagk was named chief of animal research at the German company I.G. Farben. By 1931, dyes he had been working with began to cure the illnesses in certain mice. In 1932, Domagk filed a patent for Streptozon, a red dye, and used that dye to treat a baby boy suffering from blood poisoning. The baby was cured. By 1935, Domagk was able to announce to the world the discovery of sulfa drugs, agents that could fight bacterial infection. Soon these drugs, in countless variants, were widely described as the most valuable on earth. Sulfa drugs did not kill bacteria, but they retarded their growth and gave the body a chance to jump in and finish the job.

Other antibiotics besides sulfa drugs and penicillin were devised during the following decades, and their use proliferated. The only dark side to this otherwise splendid tale of progress is that the bacteria began to fight back. Demonstrating appalling evolutionary resistance, some of the bacteria that cause gonorrhea became drug resistant. Then tuberculosis, resurgent largely because of its association with AIDS, became especially virulent. It seemed that many patients, notably among the poor, had a tendency to take their antibiotics just long enough to achieve some remission but not long enough to effect a cure. The result was that the bacteria grew strong through adversity, and drugs that once had worked very well indeed became essentially impotent.

New therapies need to be invented for these and other scourges fast. Will they come from biotechnology? Some medical researchers believe so. Already, in the 1990s, the use of gene-splicing techniques to produce new drugs has shown great promise, despite some disappointments. And the optimism for gene therapy—a pioneering approach that should soon allow doctors to correct faulty genes and prevent or remedy hereditary and other diseases—is riding a crest. Researchers around the world are striving for advances against disease on a scale and with a fervor unparalleled in the history of science. They know that medicine has plenty of reason to be proud, but they also know that this is no time for resting on laurels.

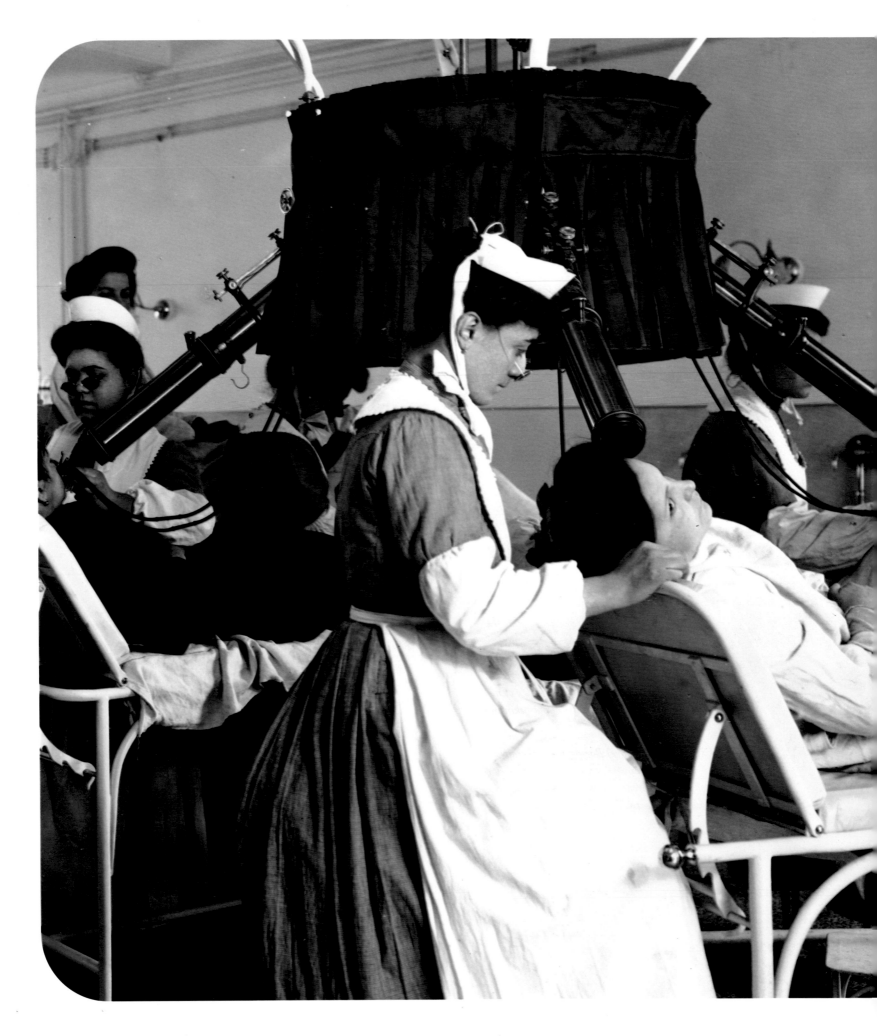

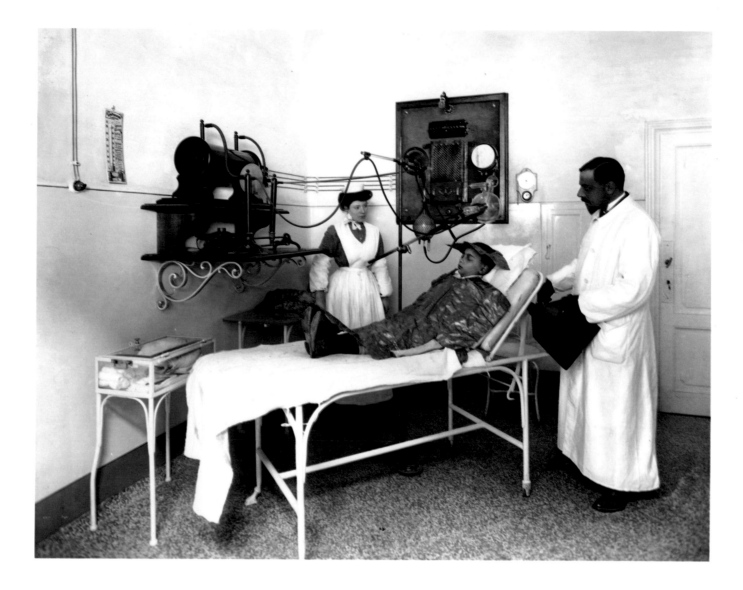

Circa 1900—*(left) The X ray soon became the darling of hospitals, drawing patients from far and wide. The X ray remained a diagnostic workhorse throughout the twentieth century, although as the century ended it was rivaled by an array of new devices for peering through the human skin into the hidden inner body.*

Circa 1900—*(above) Roentgen-ray therapy at the Institute of Fotoradiotherapy of Professor Celso Pellizzavi, Florence. X-ray therapy was to become a significant treatment for some cancers.*

The insides of our bodies, even today, seem like alien territory. When we think about ourselves at all, it is not as a fragile container full of pumping, sifting, squeezing organs. Rather, we think of our outer bodies, our appearance. In introspective moments we might reflect on our minds, but surely not on our brains. So when we find ourselves in a doctor's office and get a glimpse of the inside of our bodies in a negative or on a screen, it strikes us as magical.

Yet the ability to look directly inside the body is now anything but novel. It is, in fact, just about a hundred years old. Today the machines that peer into the body are the big cannons in the physician's arsenal, along with the computer, which insinuated itself into medical practice throughout the seventies and eighties. Today, computer programs can answer doctors' questions about an illness. Employing something called "virtual reality," the computer can "walk surgeons through" simulated but realistic procedures as though they were actually happening. And computers, preeminently, are used every day to interpret and enhance diagnostic information, making it more useful than ever before.

When the body opened up its secrets *(continued on page 164)*

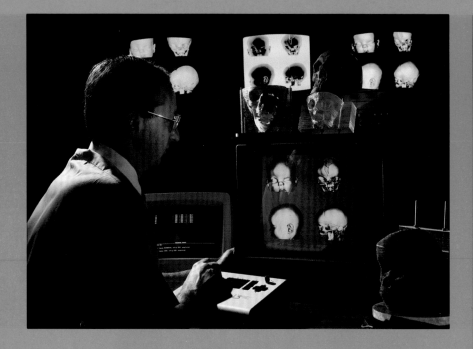

The Technology of Seeing

1988—The direct descendant of Roentgen's marvelous machine is today's CAT scanner; it's an X-ray device too, but instead of merely shooting straight on, the scanner encircles the body, to create images that are in the form of thin slices, all of them to be assembled by computer into a single, multi-dimensional image. CAT scanners are playing important roles in institutions throughout the world. This one, at the Mallincrodt Institute of Radiology at Washington University Medical Center in St. Louis, Missouri, is operated by Dr. Michael Vannier *(above)*. His eighteen-month-old patient is Lindy Chapman *(right)*, seen here entering the CAT scanning machine. Photographed by Alexander Tsiaras.

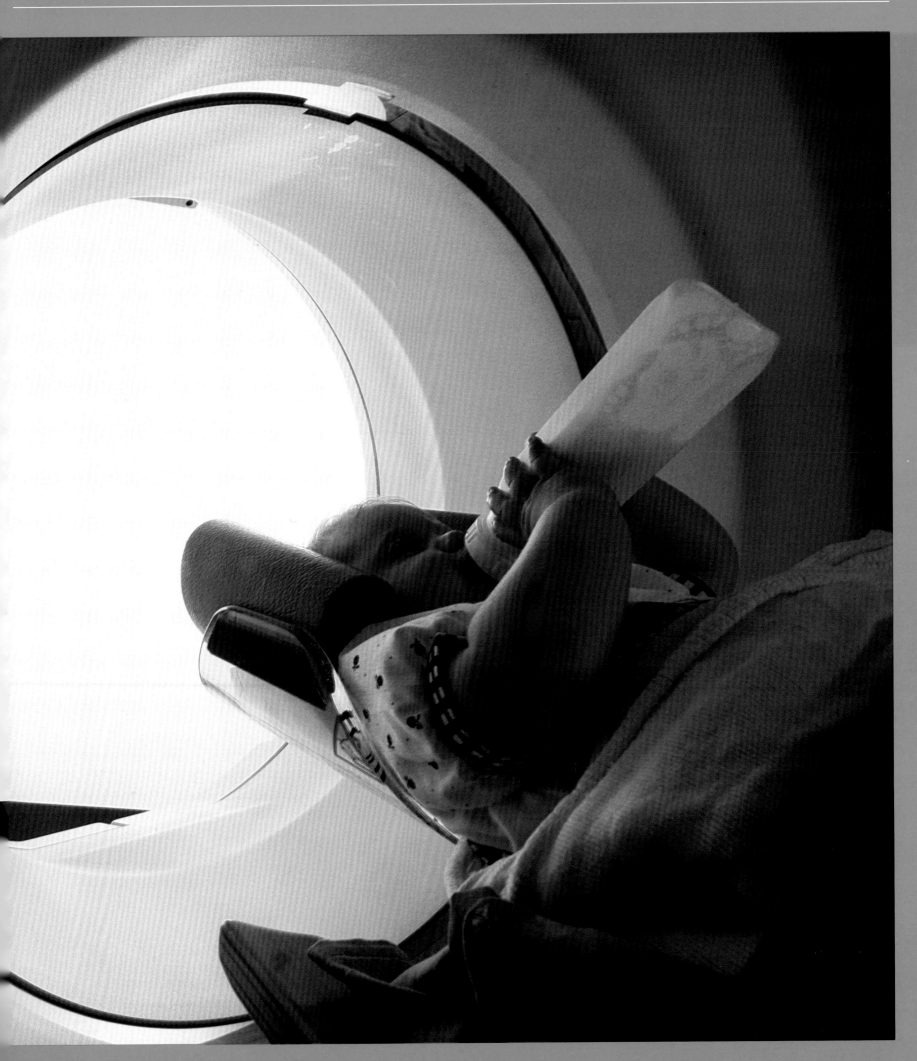

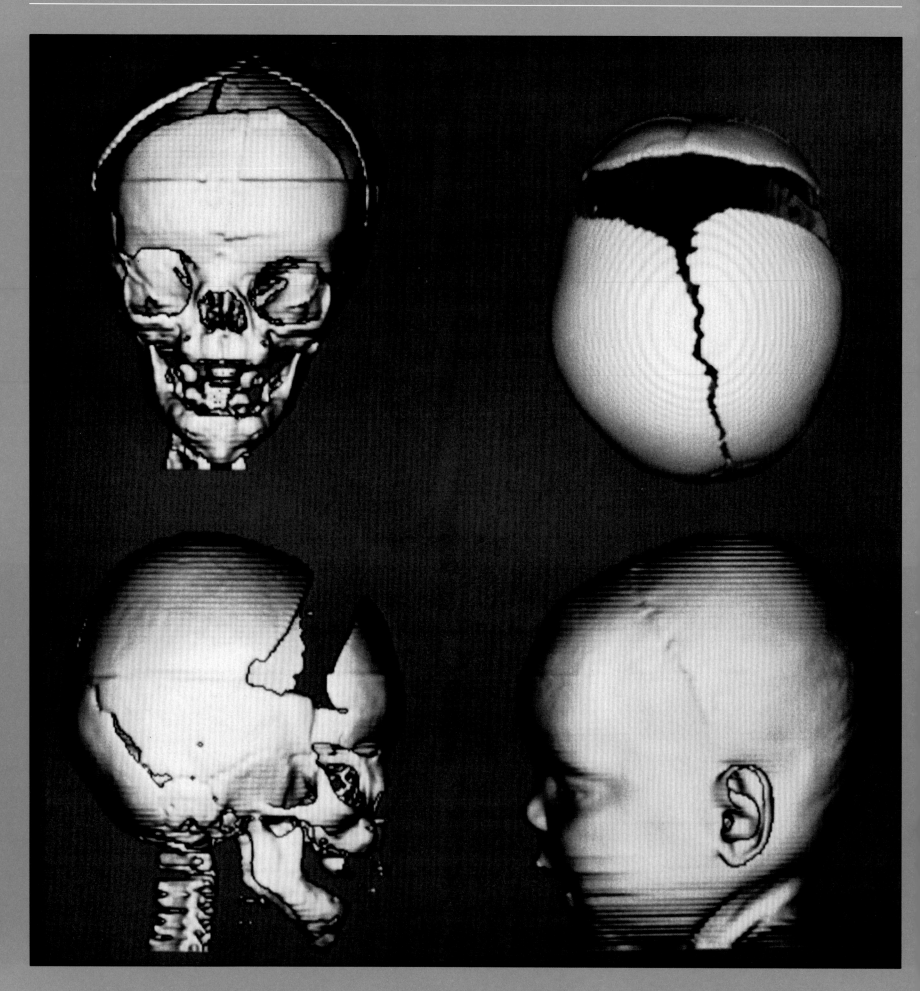

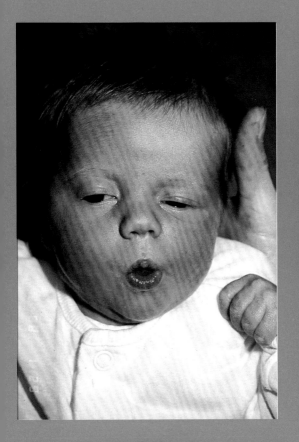

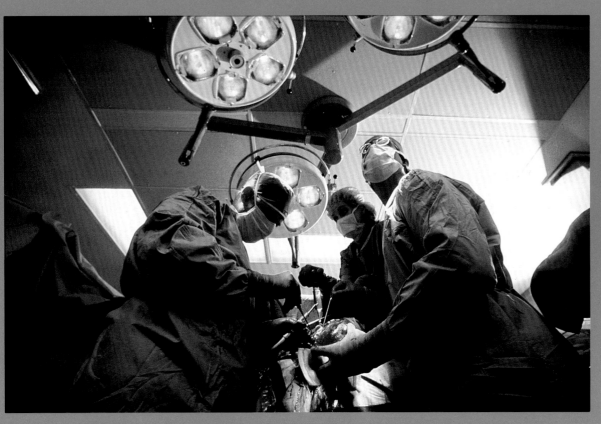

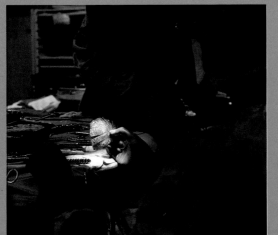

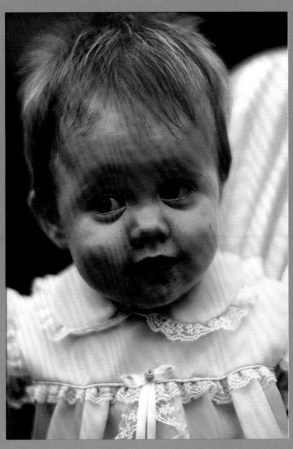

Developed in Great Britain in 1972, CAT scanners convert X-ray pictures into digital computer code to make high-resolution video images. The computer graphics employed are similar to those used to reassemble pictures beamed back from distant space probes. Depicting bone structures in detail, CAT scans can also show small differences between normal and abnormal tissues in the brain, lungs, and other organs. Three dimensional CAT images are beginning to play an important role in constructive surgery. In this series of images showing the operation in progress, the suture on the left side of Lindy Chapman's head is causing facial warping *(above, left)*. The operations to remedy Lindy's problem are performed by Jeffery Marsh *(above and far left)*. A computer generated image shows four stages of the operation *(opposite)*. Lindy is shown here after successful surgery *(left)*.

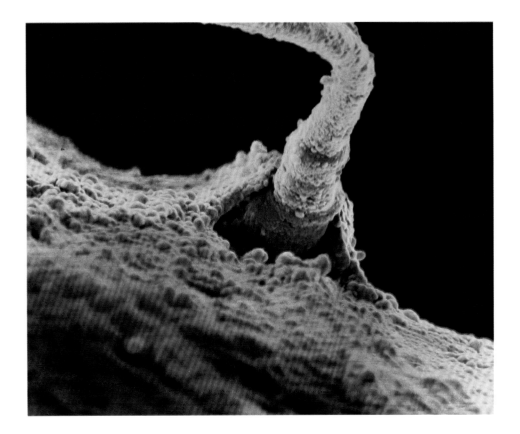

1988—*(left) The moment of conception as a sperm fertilizes an egg. Modern technology led to the formation of a new kind of medical team: the photographer and the microbiologist. Together they can see and record the body—healthy as well as sick—in greater detail than ever before. In photographs that grabbed the attention of the world when they were first published, Lennart Nilsson revealed the birth process.*

1976—*(opposite) Nilsson's photography of an embryo revealed for the first time the amazing stages of development of the human fetus. Here we see the eyes already well developed by the thirteenth week, although the lids remain closed for several months.*

in 1895 with the invention of the X ray, it followed centuries of diagnosis accomplished through interviewing the patient, making superficial observations, and listening for sounds of malfunction.

An early breakthrough was the stethoscope, conceived in 1816 in Paris by Dr. René-Théophile-Hyacinthe Laënnec, who discovered he could roll paper into a tube, put his ear at one end, and listen to an amplified sound of the heart. Like so many momentous developments, the stethoscope quickly became overinterpreted to the point where it invited mockery. But the nineteenth-century diagnostician was not only hampered by limited equipment; patients were also shy and doctors reluctant to get personal. A gynecological discussion, for instance, frequently remained on the conversational level, aided, perhaps, by a bit of tapping on the abdomen, while the body part in question went unexamined.

But in 1895, the medical darkness was illuminated by a ray of unknown nature that, because it was so mysterious, would be called an X ray. It was a November afternoon, and the German physicist Wilhelm Conrad Roentgen was experimenting with electricity. He placed a glass tube in a black paper box and then ran a current through a wire in the tube. Nearby, on a bench, he saw a faint greenish glow. But there was no beam of light in the darkened room. He ignited a match to see the room better. On the bench was a bit of cardboard coated with a phosphorescent chemical that would glow when it was struck by some kind of energy. Roentgen soon figured out that the radiation passing through the paper box onto the cardboard would also pass through other *(continued page 168)*

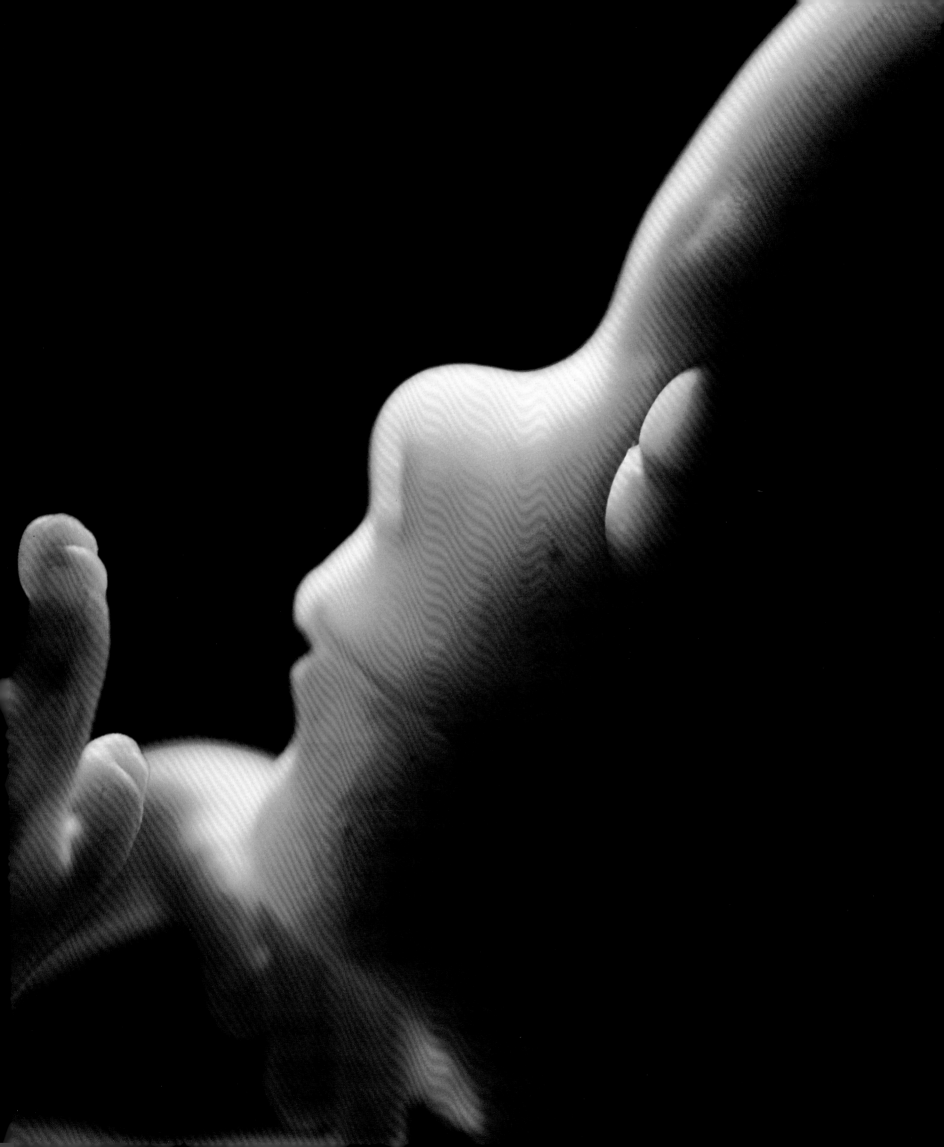

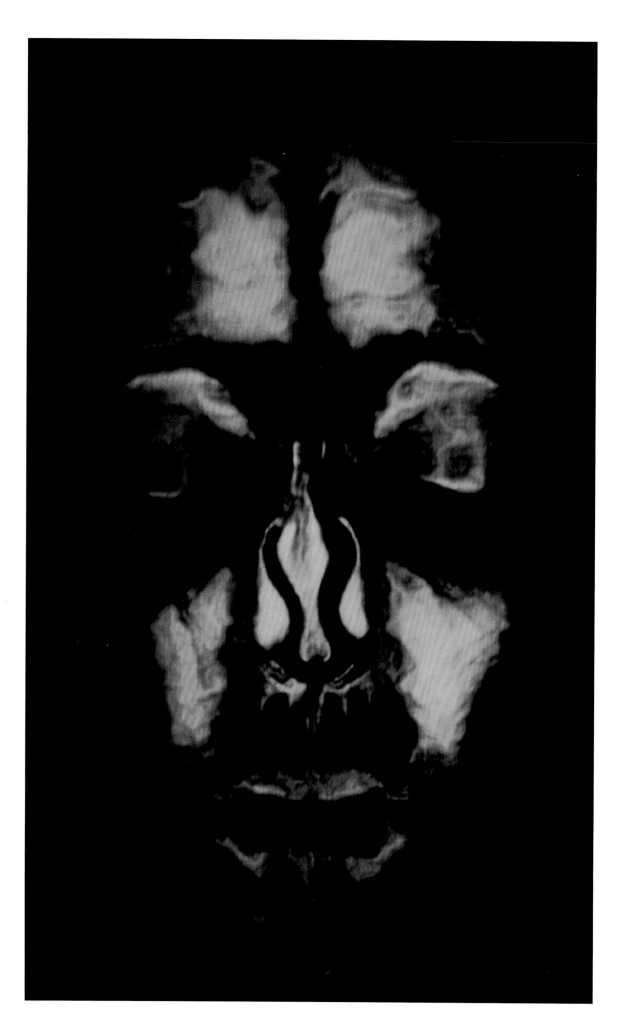

1988—*A Magnetic Resonance Imaging scan. MRI, which is frequently used to view soft tissue in high contrast, employs a combination of radio waves and a strong magnetic field. It represents a major development among the newest generation of imaging devices, which have changed the face of medicine by enabling doctors to detect problems and diseases without surgery. An important quality of MRI is that it reflects water because it focuses on the behavior of hydrogen atoms in water molecules. This allows MRI to do certain things better than CAT scanners, such as distinguishing between the brain's white matter and the water-rich gray matter. Teeth and bones, which contain little water, do not appear at all in MRI, enabling doctors to obtain a clear picture of tissues surrounding bone, such as the spinal cord. MRI has been used to spot the tiny lesions of multiple sclerosis on brain and spinal tissue. Photographed by Howard Sochurek.*

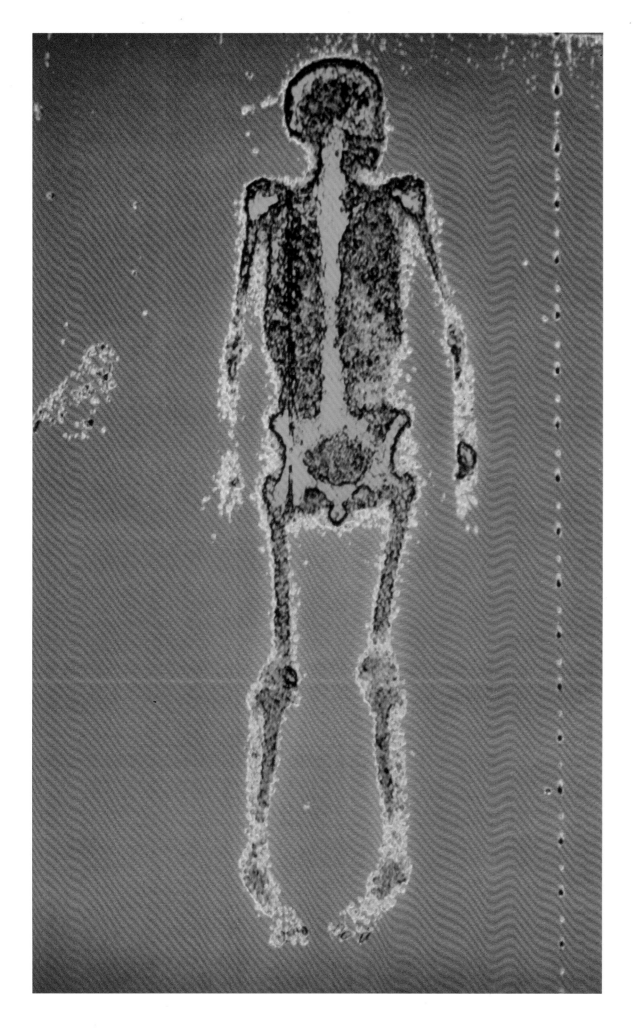

1988—The whole body is captured in a bone scan obtained using radioisotope tracers. Created by a gamma camera, the image depicts emissions of gamma rays from a phosphate tagged with technetium 99m, a low-level radioactive material. Injected into the bloodstream, the phosphate comes to rest mainly in bones, producing a comprehensive view of the skeletal system. This study was done to determine whether or not cancer had spread to the bones from a tumor in the breast of a fifty-six-year-old woman, and proved it had not. Photographed by Howard Sochurek.

things—wood, porous matter, even some metal. When his hand moved into the radiation's line, to his astonishment he saw the shadows of his bones on the phosphorescent screen. The radiation had evidently passed right through his skin and flesh.

Soon, Roentgen was able to send off a paper to the Würzburg Physical Medical Society, entitling it "On a New Kind of Ray." By January 1896 he was lecturing on the discovery and the whole world was discussing it. Shortly thereafter came the invention of the fluoroscope, which was actually a kind of throwback to Roentgen's first experience. Instead of using a photographic plate to capture a still image, it employed a screen coated with a fluorescent chemical allowing observation of the moving skeleton of a body.

The X ray's impact was incalculable, augmenting the less precise signals supplied by touch and sound. Now a physician could see exactly where a bone was broken or find a foreign object (a bullet, for example) embedded deep in the body. The discovery was so unexpected and so incredible that many contemporaries had a hard time truly comprehending the experience. As researchers came to better understand how X rays worked, passing through some materials more readily than others, they continued to refine the technology. About 1896, Walter B. Cannon of Harvard began an investigation that ultimately would lead to the less than delightful experience (as anyone knows who's had it) called the "lower G.I. series." Cannon started to work with a substance called bismuth, which, when swallowed, facilitated pictures of the gastrointestinal system.

This was a dizzying time for diagnostic innovation of all sorts. The electrocardiograph, initially explored in Germany in the late nineteenth century, was refined in the early twentieth by a Dutch physiologist, Willem Einthoven. Other evidence of illness never seen before was suddenly coming into clear view. The German physician and microscopy pioneer Robert Koch found in 1882 that tuberculosis was caused by bacteria, a breakthrough of inestimable significance. By the twentieth century, the high-powered microscope had achieved its position as a premier tool in the search for evidence of a disease, and the laboratory became a necessary adjunct to the craft of the practicing physician.

In the latter part of the twentieth century, Roentgen's X ray still functions as a diagnostic workhorse, though developments are afoot that greatly amplify its usefulness and that provide even better viewing of organs through spectacularly different techniques.

In the late sixties in Britain, a future Nobel Prize was in the wings. An electrical engineer, Godfrey Hounsfield, was at work on the machine that would become the Computerized Axial Tomography (CAT) scanner. South African-American physicist Allan Cormack developed the necessary mathematical formulations for the device. The idea of the CAT scan, which would be a functioning reality by 1972, was essentially to surround the body by an X-ray tube that produces a picture revealing a thin slice so that,

1988—*(opposite) This three-dimensional line drawing of the shape of the human head, displayed as if in a contour map, is the product of data drawn from a CAT scan. This image reveals a brain tumor of the right ventricle. The shape of the tumor emerges in green, with the ventricles colored purple. The eyes appear in red. Photographed by Philippe Plailly.*

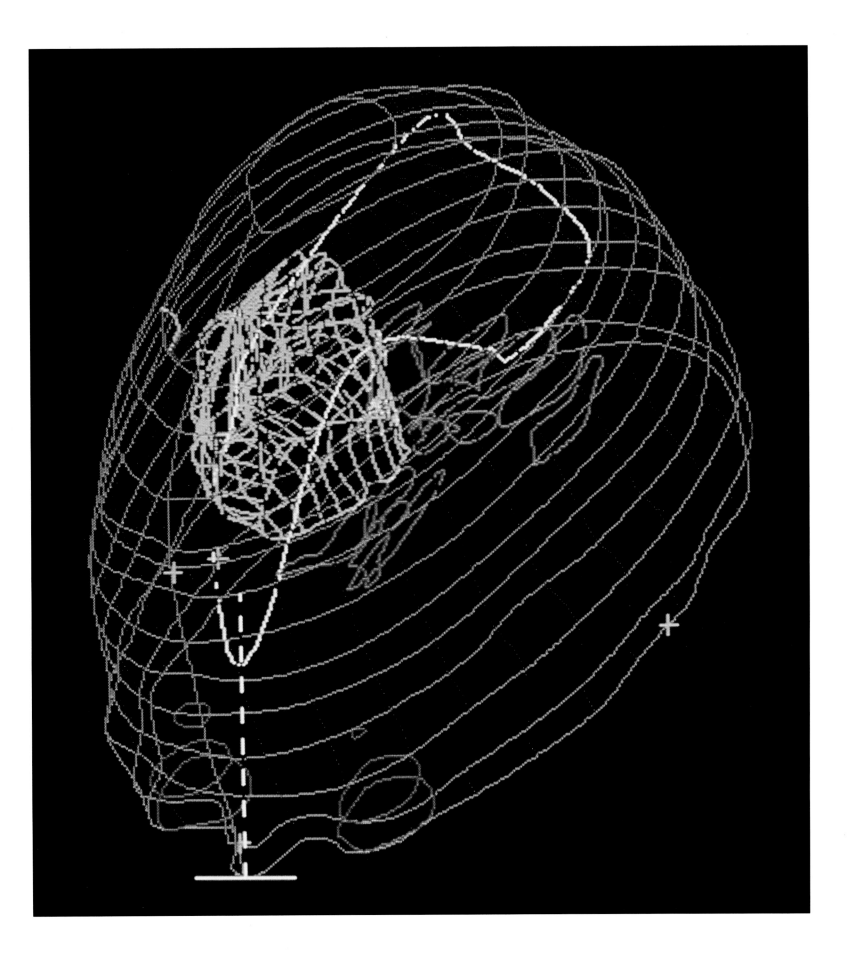

instead of looking at the body head-on, one sees a cross-section. A series of these images could then be assembled by computer into a single, three-dimensional view of bones, muscle, and organs.

By the 1980s, rival technologies proliferated, including the magnetic resonance imaging (MRI) machine and in the 1990s, major new devices including the Positron Emission Tomography (PET) scanner, which is able to provide a view of the biochemical functioning of body parts in action, as well as their structure.

The magnetic resonance imaging (MRI) machine, for instance, can also peer into the body (though at incredibly high cost, with a single examination running as much as $15,000). Magnetic resonance imaging is slower than CAT scanning (thirty to forty-five minutes, compared to just two or three seconds) but does not need to bombard the tissues with radiation to obtain a picture. This technique employs an immensely powerful magnet—so powerful that it might dislodge metal inside the body, which means that patients with metal plates or pacemakers have to stay away.

Ultrasound has become a primary tool in medicine, especially in the examination of fetuses in the womb. As the century ends, this and other advanced devices are leading physicians into stunning new areas of accomplishment, among them the ability to operate on an unborn baby in the womb. They can see so well into the mother's body that when they spot trouble—such as excess fluid in the brain of the fetus—they can move to remedy it with tiny surgical implements. Some medical tools in the future will be so tiny that they will be perceptible to the eye only through a microscope. Electronic sensors that fit on the end of a wire as thin as a fishing line are already available. Doctors can send such a sensor through a vein to the heart, where it is capable of making blood-pressure readings to a degree of sensitivity unheard-of previously. Another use for sensors (though like many cutting-edge applications this is still in the future) involves a two-pronged hypodermic needle with sensor mounted on one tine, and a tiny light bulb on the opposing needle tip: tumors can be detected by measuring the light that passes from the microbulb through tissue to the sensor. And one day soon, miniature rotary motors will be so small and fine that they can saw away cataracts on the eye. The know-how for making these tools is already well advanced; some of the most creative minds in medical science are defining the role of microdevices for the twenty-first century.

INTO THE FUTURE

R eaching for the millennium, we can no longer approach medicine with the blind faith of the past. Today's health care is too complicated for that, and we know too much about its limitations. At the same time, there is every reason to feel the deepest appreciation for medicine's accomplishments. The capacity of modern medicine to heal, to extend life, has become so great that it hardly seems possible that a mere hundred years could have witnessed it all.

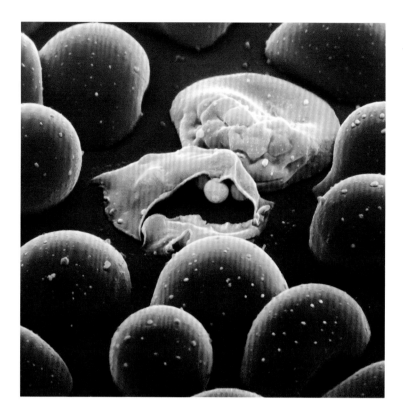

1980—(above) Red blood cell ruptured by invading malarial plasmodia.
Photographed by Lennart Nilsson.

1991—(opposite) AIDS has been the most controversial medical issue of the late twentieth century. Working with Maureen Mangiardi of Creative Media Concepts, the computer artist, Regina Tierney, interpreted data from magnetic resonance imaging and the electron microscope to create a visual rendering of the HIV virus. The virus attacks the much larger T-cell, a key defender employed by the immune system. Both virus and T-cell are represented in their exact proportions. Holograms, three-dimensional imaging, and virtual reality have informed a new generation of artists and doctors alike, as tools such as the electron microscope and MRI create windows on the limitless expanse of inner worlds.

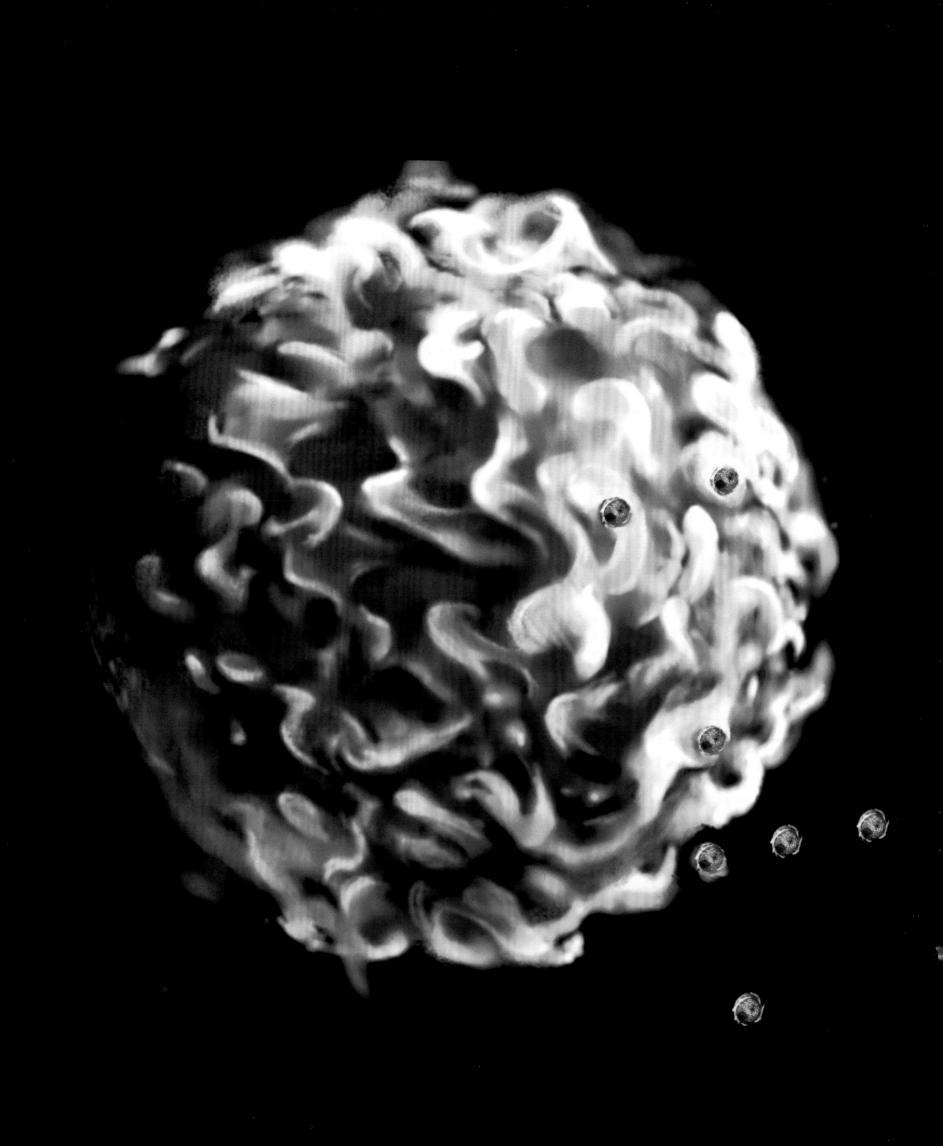

CREDITS

Rick Smolan and Phillip Moffitt, *Creators*

Charles Melcher and Nicholas Callaway, *Producers*

Nan Richardson and Catherine Chermayeff, *Project Editors, Umbra Editions, Inc.*

Thomas K. Walker, *Art Director and Designer, GRAF/x*

True Sims, *Production Manager*

Eulalia Herrero Salas, *Associate Editor, Umbra Editions, Inc.*

Sherri Whitmarsh, *Design Assistant, GRAF/x*

Cheryl MacLachlan, *Director of Sponsorships*

Preston Williams, *Sponsorship Marketing Director*

Thomas West and George Leonard, *Consulting Editors*

Dr. Allan E. Dumont, *Professor Emeritus of Surgery, New York University, Medical Advisor*

Aaron Schindler, *Photo Contest Director*

Ivan Wong, Toshiya Masuda, *Production Associates*

Martha Lazar, Chris Noble, Denise Rocco, Sheila Schat, *Editorial Assistants*

Tanya Wright, *Fact Checker*

Barbara Bergeron, *Copy Editor*

Mary Susan MacAverey, *Photo Contest Assistant*

Picture Researchers

Susan Duca, *Consulting Editor*

Stuart Alexander

Michael Clapp

Claudine Doury

Mary Dunkin

Birgitta Forsell

Susan Friedman

Jane Marsching

Dan McManus

Karen Moller

Eithne Richardson

Margaret Sidlovsky

George Slade

Danica Suskin

ABOUT THIS BOOK

Medicine's Great Journey was set in Adobe Garamond and Trajan typefaces. Thomas Palmer made the 300-line separations for the black and white duotones. Laserscan of Phoenix, Arizona prepared the 200-line, four-color separations. The book was printed by Universal Press, Providence, Rhode Island.

ACKNOWLEDGMENTS

This book was produced from a host of archives, including hospitals, museums, historical societies, and private collections, the work of individual photographers and photo agencies, as well as the files of companies active in the field of medicine. Images were collected from over six hundred sources around the world, notably France, Germany, Switzerland, Canada, Italy, England, Sweden, Russia, and Australia. Over a dozen talented researchers, all experts in their fields, exerted themselves to uncover exceptional, rare, and, in some cases, never-before-seen photographs. We are grateful to them for their professionalism and grace under pressure. The decision process was an exceptionally difficult one, and many fascinating photographs eventually—and regretfully—were excluded. The nearly two hundred images in the finished book represent a diverse and astonishing version of medicine's history as depicted in photography.

None of this would have been possible without the very generous advice, patience, cooperation, and guidance of a number of individuals and institutions. We would like to acknowledge them below, on behalf of all those involved in making this book, in alphabetical order, and to extend again our heartfelt thanks and gratitude for their support.

Major Sponsors

Olympus Corporation

Health Magazine

Light Source Computer Imaging, Inc.

Eastman Kodak Company

Institutions

ABC-TV 20/20 News

Actuel

Adobe Systems

Afro-American Historical and Cultural Museum

Agence Vu

Aldus Corporation

AMA Medical News

American Cancer Society

American Express

American Lung Association

American Red Cross

Amon Carter Museum

Apple Computer Inc.

Apple Singapore

Art Institute of Chicago

Arts & Communication Counselors

Atwater Kent Museum

Balestra Capital

Bellevue Hospital

Bettmann Archive

Big Idea Group

Black Star

Body Shop International

Bristol-Myers Squibb

Brown Brothers

Buffalo and Erie County Historical Society

Burns Archive

Woodfin Camp and Associates

Canadian Centre for Architecture

Cathay Pacific Airways Ltd.

CE Software

Cedar Rapids Gazette

Center for Creative Imaging

Center for Creative Photography

Center for the Study of Nursing, University of Pennsylvania

Centers for Disease Control

Children's Hospital of Philadelphia

Chrysler Museum

Cincinnati Historical Society

City of Edmonton Archive

City of Milwaukee Health Department

Collins San Francisco

Contact Press Images

Francis A. Countway Library of Medicine, Harvard University

Cowan Liebovitz & Latman

Creative Media Concepts

Culver Pictures

Cunningham Communications

DDB Needham Worldwide Advertising

Dinkelspiel, Donovan & Reder

Sheila Donnelly & Associates

Duke University

Eastman Kodak Company

Europress

F-D-C Reports

FPG International

Fratelli Alinari

Free Library of Philadelphia

Frontier Nursing Service Inc.

General Magic

GEO Magazine, New York

Georgia Department of Archives and History

German Red Cross

J. Paul Getty Museum

Global Village Communication

Grey Art Gallery

Gunderson Clinic

Hartford Medical Society

Harvard University

Hewlett Packard

Highland Hospital

Hippocrates Partners

Hospital for
  Sick Children
Hulton Picture
  Company
Idaho Historical Society
Imagine Films
Imagineworks
Indiana University
Institute for the Future
International Museum
  of Photography
  at George Eastman
  House
International Red Cross
  Museum
Iowa State University
Johns Hopkins Medical
  Institutions
C. G. Jung Foundation
  of New York
Kansas Historical
  Society
Keystone
Lawrence Lane
Life Picture Sales
Light Source Computer
  Imaging, Inc.
Magnum Photos,
  New York
Magnum Photos, Paris
March of Dimes

Mary Ellen Mark Library
Maryland Historical
  Society
Massachusetts General
  Hospital
McCalls
Médecins sans Frontières
Medtronic
Menninger Hospital
Merck & Company
Metis
Micronet
Edward G. Miner
  Library, University
  of Rochester
Minnesota Art Institute
Minnesota Historical
  Society
Missouri School
  of Journalism
Montana Historical
  Society
Montefiore Medical
  Center
Mount Sinai Hospital
Municipal Archives of
  the City of New York
Musée de l'Elysée
Museum of the City
  of New York
Mutter Museum

National Geographic
  Society
National Institutes
  of Health
Nebraska State
  Historical Society
New Haven Historical
  Society
New-York Historical
  Society
New York Hospital-
  Cornell Medical
  Center
New York Times
Newsweek Magazine
NeXT
Northwestern University
Novo Nordisk
Ohio Historical Society
Ohio State University
Olympus Corporation
Pallas Photo
Parke-Davis
Pennsylvania Hospital
People Magazine
Photo Researchers, Inc.
Photographers Aspen
Piper, Jaffray &
  Hopwood
Proskauer Rose, Goetz
  & Mendelsohn

Purdue University
QMS Inc.
Rapho
Release 1.0
Republic of Tea
Rockefeller University
Rush-Presbyterian-
  St. Luke's Medical
  Center
St. Paul Pioneer Press
San Jose Mercury News
Schering-Plough
  Corporation
Showtime Networks Inc.
Smithsonian Institution
Sophia Smith Collec-
  tion, Smith College
Sports Illustrated
State Historical Society
  of Wisconsin
Staten Island Historical
  Society
Stern Magazine
Sun Venture
  Travel Systems
Supermac Technology
Sygma Photo News
Time Warner Inc.
Transglobe
Tulip Films
University of Alberta

University of Kentucky
University of Louisville
University of Minnesota
University of Oklahoma
Userland Software
Utne Reader
Westlight
World Health
  Organization
Yale University
  Medical Library

Individuals
Rhoda and Ira Albom
John Alfano
Andy Anderson
Jane Anderson
Wayne Anderson
Jack Angel
Matthew Antezzo
Diana Arecco
Bill Atkinson
Fran Antmann
Dr. Raymond Bahar
Linda Bailey
Sharon Bailey
Gordon Baldwin
Dr. James Balog
Teri Barbero
Allen Barr
Catherine Bassney

Suzelle Baudouin
Terry Bean
Frank Becher
Douglas Beckham
David Beezley
David Bell
Mary Bell
Janie Joseland Bennett
Richard Bernstein
David Biehn
Michele Biondi
Jesse Birnbaum
Christophe Blaser
Amy Bonetti
Shirley Bonnem
Jessica Brackman
Sid Braginsky
Paul Brainerd
Jo Anne Branham
Russell Brown
Dr. Shirley Brown
Scott Brownstein
Rudy Bryce
Lucinda Burkepile
Kelly E. Burnet
Dr. Stanley Burns
James Busby
Victor Byrd
Woodfin Camp
Stuart Campbell
John E. Carter

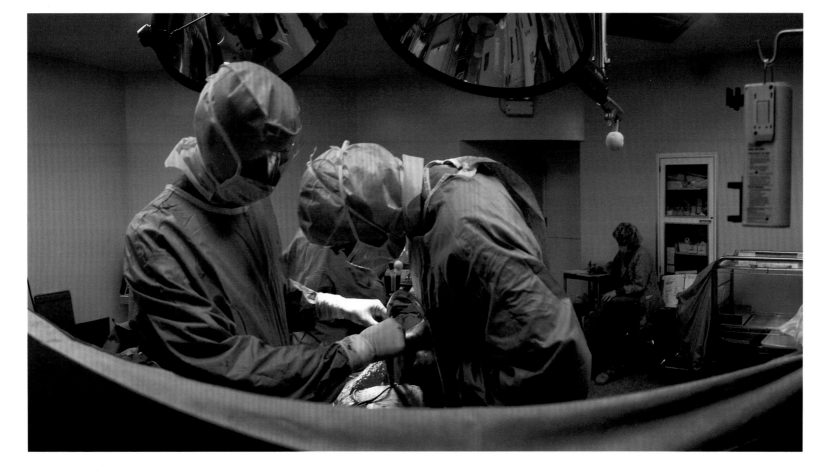

Denise Caruso
Carla Castillo
May Castleberry
Dr. Frank Catchpool
Christian Caujolle
Mike and Gina Cerre
Cathy Cesario
Satjiv Chahill
Howard Chapnick
Albert Chu
Dan Church
Randy Churner
Sarah Clarke
Kenneth Cobb
Don Conklin
Rob Cook
Guy Cooper
Alessandra Corti
Elisabeth J. Cox
Angelica Cu
Andie Cunningham
Jonathan David
Anne Day
Kate de Castlebajac
Melissa Dehncke
Chris DeMoulin
Ray DeMoulin
Lou Desiderio
Laura DeYoung
Herman Diettering
Byron Dobell
Sheila Donnelly
Arnold Drapkin
Gene and Gayle
    Driskell
Natasha Driskell
Jana Drvota
John Durniak

Esther Dyson
Oscar Dystell
Ruth Eichhorn
Sandra Eisert
Kristin Ellison
Ellen Erwitt
Elloitt Erwitt
Jennifer Erwitt
Robert Eskind
Wendy Ewald
Tibor Farcas
Harlan Felt
Dominique Fisher
Patricia Fleming
Doris Fong
Francis Fralen
Marie-Agnes Gainon
Liz Gallin
Marvin and Leslie Gans
Sharon Garrett
Ivan Garzon
Jean-Pierre Gaume
Noreen Geistle
Ron Gentile
Barbara Gibson
Diane Gilday
Suzanne Goldstein
Robert Goldwin
Dr. Fred Gorelick
Tauny Graham
Brian Grazer
Susan Grigg
John Gruhlke
Claus Guglberger
Steve Guttman
Ferenc Gyorgye
Stephan Hagen
Dr. Joseph Harb

Richard Heckler
Dr. David Heiden
Dr. Joseph Henderson
Lilith Hendrickson
Barbara Henley
Phillip Herres
Andy Hertzfeld
James Higa
Dominique Hoefflin
Chris Hollern
Christine Hollings
June Honey
Elizabeth Hooks
Christopher Hoolihan
Thomas House
Ron Howard
Say Hutchinson
Charles and Carol Isaacs
Matthew Isenburg
Rita Jacobs
Paul Jansen
Brooks Johnson
Kirk Johnson
Barbara Jones
Becky Jordan
Cindy Joyce
Nicola Kamens
Susan Kare
Andy Karsch
Ruth Kasloff
Joan Keith
Tom Kennedy
Lorinda Klein
Kent Kobersteen
Rebecca Kohl
Hans Krause, Jr.
Andy Krausharr
Ellen Kunes
Bill Kuykendall
Eliane and J. P. Laffont
Jane LaMantia
Sonia Land
Elke Langmaack-
    Scheiber
Margaret Lavin
George Leonard
Adele Lerner
Carol Judy Leslie
Dorothy Levenson
Martin Levin
Jonathan Levine
Gerard Levy
John Loengard
Ernest Lofblad
John Lovett
Cecile Lucas
John Maglione
Alfred Mandel
Maureen Mangiardi
Michelle E. Marcella

Karen Marta
Claudine Maugendre
Jim Mauzey
Stewart McBride
Georgia McCabe
Barbara McCandless
Lucretia McClure
Kerry McGrath
Jim Melcher
Doug and Teresa
    Menuez
Nadine Merryman
Gail Miller
Dan Mjolsness
Brenda Moffitt
Caroline Morris
Jacqui Mott
Karen Mullarkey
Linda Neumann
Diane Newman
Dianne Nilsen
Mrs. Lennart Nilsson
Julie Nolan
Barbara Norfleet
Peter Norman
Jean-Christophe
    Nothias
Linda O'Donnell
Karen Olcott
John O'Neil
Dr. Mario Orlandi
Dr. Dean Ornish
Gene Ostroff
Rusty Pallas
Wendy Palmer
Daniel Paul
Douglas Peckmann
Gabe Perle
William Perry
Christian Peterson
Klaus Plarmann
Tess Platt
Françoise Ponnet
Mary Ann Price
Jeff Pruss
Eric Pumroy
Jill Quasha
Pat Quinn
Mark Raff
Arian D. Ravanbakhsh
Pamela Reed
Sharon Reed
Thomas P. Reilly
Spencer Reiss
Patti Richards
Martha Richardson
Diane Riley
Ty Roberts
Justin and Debby
    Robinson

Anita Roddick
Marge Romano
Joan Rosenberg
Bill, Faye, and Sam
    Rosenzweig
Kathy Ryan
Paul Saffo
Nola Safro
Rita Scaglia
Kathy Scheiner
Eric Schrier
John Sculley
Steve Seekins
Tom Sellars
Harold Shain
John Sheehy
Ron Simms
Julie Sims
Agnes Sire
Bob Siroka
Richard Skeie
Jeffrey Smith
Joe Smith
Megan Smith
Rick Smith
Rodney Smith
Leslie Smolan
Marvin and Gloria
    Smolan
Sandy and Reed
    Smolan
Myra Smoot
Dr. Alan Solomon
Joy and Marty
    Solomon
Mike Solomon
Sandy Sonnessa
Christie Stanley
Dieter Steiner
Robert Stevens
David Stout
Laura Strauss
David Strettell
Jeff Sturchio
Jung Suh
Peter Sutch
Lena Tabori
Harri Taranto
Joe Tartt
Michael Tchao
Fred Telling
Paul Theroux
Scott Thode
Mark Thompson
Holger Thoss
Regina Tierney
Eric and Nina Utne
John and Marva Warnock
Marion Wedekind
Margaret Welch

Dr. Charles Wells
David White
Fred Wilkinson
Dave Willard
Dorothy Williams
Hazel Williams
Dave Winer
Sylvia Wolf
Richard Wolfe
Michelle Wong
Gretchen Worden
Simon Worrin
Nina Kaiden Wright
Richard Saul Wurman
Dawn Wyman
Eric Zarakov
Dela Zitkus

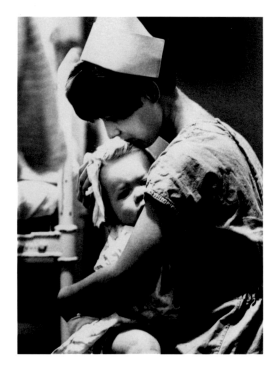

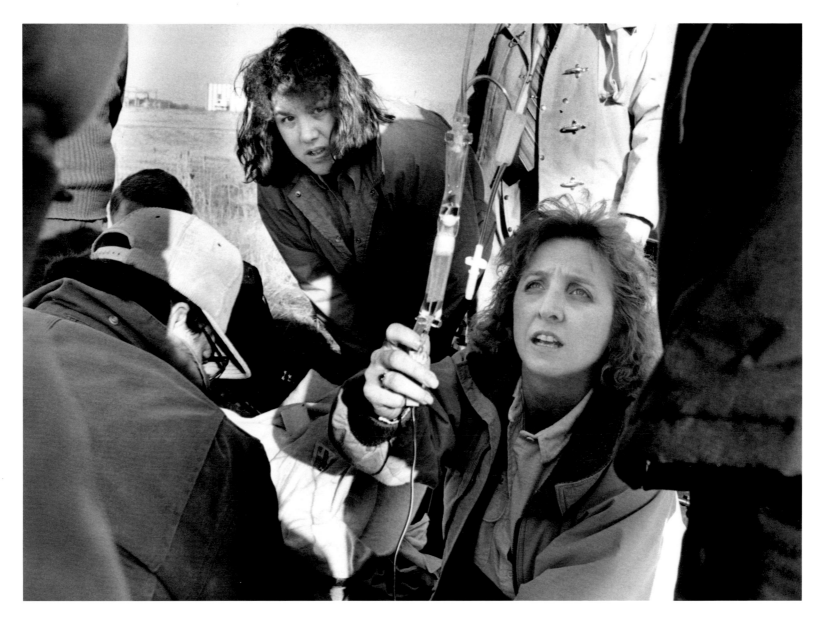

Picture Credits

COVER: W. Eugene Smith, Black Star
BACK COVER: L. C. Dillon, Courtesy Stanley B. Burns, M.D., and The Burns Archive
ii-iii Photographer unknown, Courtesy Rush-Presbyterian-St. Luke's Medical Center Archives
iv-v © Luc Choquer/Metis
vi-vii David Joel, Courtesy Rush-Presbyterian-St. Luke's Medical Center Archives
viii-ix Edouard Boubat, © Agence Top
6-7 Photographer unknown, Collection of the Maryland Historical Society, Baltimore
8-9 Photographer unknown, Culver Pictures
10 Photographer unknown, Brown Brothers
11(top) Photographer unknown, © ADN GmbH Bildarchiv
11(bottom) Photographer unknown, Musée de l'Elysée, Lausanne
12 R. H. Lawrence, courtesy of The New-York Historical Society, N.Y.C.

13 Photographer unknown, Urban Archives, Temple University
14-15 Lewis Hine, International Museum of Photography at George Eastman House
16-17 Photographer unknown, Municipal Archives, Department of Records and Information Services, City of New York
17 (top) Department of Public Works Official Photographer, City Archives of Philadelphia: Bureau of Health
18 Photographer unknown, California Museum of Photography, Keystone-Mast Collection, University of California
19 Photographer unknown, Brown Brothers
20-21 Photographer unknown, Iowa State University Library/University Archives
21 (top) Photographer unknown, Roger Viollet
22-25 Photographer unknown, Archives, The Hospital for Sick Children, Toronto
26 A. T. Beals, Bellevue Hospital Center Archives
27 Tom Merryman, Cedar Rapids Gazette
28-29 Photographer unknown, State Historical Society of Wisconsin

29 (top) Photographer unknown, Culver Pictures
30-31 Photographer unknown, Francis A. Countway Library of Medicine, Harvard University
32 Albert Fenn, *Life* Magazine © Time Warner Inc.
33 Alfred Eisenstaedt, *Life* Magazine © Time Warner Inc.
34 Photographer unknown, © Keystone
35 (top) Photographer unknown, © Keystone
35 (bottom) Photographer unknown, Ekstrom Library, Photographic Archives, University of Louisville
36-37 J. L. Courtinat, © Rapho
38-39 Anders Petersen, © MIRA Bildarchiv
40-41 Bernard Bisson, © Sygma
42-43 Max Thorek, International Museum of Photography at George Eastman House
44 Hermann Krone, Société Française de la Photographie
45 Photographer unknown, Courtesy Stanley B. Burns, M.D., and The Burns Archive
46-47 Photographer unknown, Museum of the City of New York, The Byron Collection

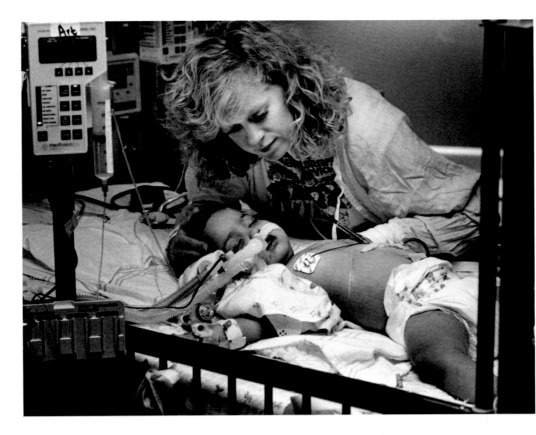

47 (top) Courtesy Dr. Michael Duff, Rolla, Missouri

48-49 Southworth and J. J. Hawes,
The Massachusetts General Hospital Archives

49 (top) Photographer unknown, The Francis A.
Countway Library of Medicine,
Harvard University

50 (top) W. H. Willard Jones, Bettmann Archive

50-51 Photographer unknown, © Keystone

52-53 Photographer unknown, Collection Centre
Canadien d'Architecture/Canadian Centre
for Architecture, Montreal

53 (top), 54-55 Photographer unknown,
Harvey Cushing-John Hay Whitney
Medical Library, Yale University

56-57 Photographer unknown, Archives,
The Hospital for Sick Children, Toronto

57 (top) Photographer unknown, Courtesy of The
Atwater Kent Museum

58-59 Photographer unknown, Bellevue Hospital
Archives

59 (top) Photographer unknown, New Haven
Historical Society

60-61 (bottom) Photographer unknown,
Bellevue Hospital Archives

61 (top) Photographer unknown, Museum of the
City of New York, The Byron Collection

62 (top) Photographer unknown, Archives,
The Hospital for Sick Children, Toronto

62-63 Photographer unknown, Minnesota Historical
Society

64 Photographer unknown, © Keystone

65 (top) Photographer unknown, Bellevue Hospital
Archives

65 (bottom) Photographer unknown, New York

Hospital-Cornell Medical Center

66 (top) Photographer unknown, Courtesy Stanley B.
Burns, M.D., and The Burns Archive

66 (bottom) Photographer unknown, Western History
Collections, University of Oklahoma Library

67 Photographer unknown, New York Hospital-
Cornell Medical Center and
Michael Leitman, M.D.

68-69 Photographer unknown, Courtesy of the
Edward G. Miner Library, Rochester, N.Y.

70-73 Alfred Eisenstaedt, *Life* Magazine
© Time Warner Inc.

74 Ritake, Urban Archives, Temple University,
Philadelphia, Pennsylvania

75 Photographer unknown, © Keystone

76-77 Thomas Stephan/Christoph &
Mayer Fotoarchiv

78 George Krause

79 Jean-Philippe Charbonnier, © Agence Top

80-81 Wenil Field, © Rapho

82 (top) Elsburgh Clarke

82-83 Andy Levin

84-85 (top) Eugene Richards, © 1989 Magnum
Photos Inc., from *The Knife and Gun Club* by
Eugene Richards with permission of
The Atlantic Monthly Press

86 Photographer unknown, Courtesy of
the Library of Congress

87 (top) Photographer unknown, The Massachusetts
General Hospital Archives

87 (bottom) Walter Willard Boyd, Harvey Cushing-
John Hay Whitney Medical Library,
Yale University

88 (top) Photographer unknown, Brown Brothers

88 (bottom) Photographer unknown, © Roger
Viollet

89 (top left) Photographer unknown, Harvey
Cushing-John Hay Whitney Medical Library,
Yale University

89 (top right) Millborne of Aylesbury, Wellcome
Institute Library, London

89 (bottom) Photographer unknown,
© Archiv Interfoto

90-91 Photographer unknown, © Keystone

92-93 Photographer unknown, Center for the
Study of the History of Nursing, School of
Nursing, University of Pennsylvania

93 (top) Photographer unknown, The Alan Mason
Chesney Medical Archives of the Johns
Hopkins Medical Institutions

94-95 Photographer unknown, New York Hospital-
Cornell Medical Center

96-97 W. Eugene Smith, © Black Star

98-99 Laura Gilpin, © Amon Carter Museum,
Fort Worth, Texas, Laura Gilpin Archives

99 (top) Arthur Rothstein, Courtesy of the
Library of Congress

100-101 Photographer unknown,
American Red Cross

102 Russell Lee, Courtesy of the Library
of Congress

103 Hansel Mieth, *Life* Magazine
© Time Warner Inc.

104-107 W. Eugene Smith, © Black Star

108-109 Photographer unknown, Joseph W.
Stilwell Collection, Hoover Institution
Archives, Stanford University

109 (top) Photographer unknown, Collection
International Red Cross and Red Crescent
Museum (MICR), Geneva. Photographic print
courtesy of the Red Cross and Red Crescent
Societies Alliance, Moscow. All rights reserved.

109 (top) Photographer unknown,
Press Illustrating Services Inc.

110 (top) Robert Capa, © Magnum Photos Inc.

110-111 Photographer unknown, Culver Pictures

112-113 (top) Photographer unknown,
American Red Cross

114-115 Photographer unknown, Culver Pictures

115 (top) Photographer unknown, Deutsches Rotes
Kreuz, Generalsekretariat

116-119 W. Eugene Smith, © Black Star

120 John Dominus, *Life* Magazine
© Time Warner Inc.

121 Mary Ellen Mark, © Mary Ellen Mark Library

122 (top) Raymond Depardon,
© Magnum Photos Inc.

122-123 Marion Kaplan,
© 1978 National Geographic Society

124-127 Misha Erwitt, © Magnum Photos Inc.

128 David Heiden

129 Alfred Eisenstaedt, *Life* Magazine
© Time Warner Inc.

130-131, 132 (top) Photographer unknown,

Fratelli Alinari

132-133 Photographer unknown, Collection Centre Canadien d'Architecture/Canadian Centre for Architecture, Montreal

134-135 Photographer unknown, National Archives, photo no. 90-G-128-3

135 (top) Lennart Nilsson, © *Behold Man,* Little, Brown and Company

136 Nathan Benn, © Woodfin Camp

137 Annie Griffiths Belt

138-139 William Strode-HUMANA

139 (top) Bill Luster, © Matrix

140-141 Fred Ward, © Black Star

141 (top) Lennart Nilsson

142 Lynn Johnson, © Black Star

143 Charles O'Rear, © Westlight

144 (bottom) © I.P.L. Australia

144-145 Alexander Tsiaras

146-147 Photographer unknown, Bettmann Archive

147 (top) Photographer unknown, © Keystone

147 (bottom) Photographer unknown,

Courtesy Rush-Presbyterian-St.Luke's Medical Center Archives

148 Photographer unknown, © Rapho

149 Gordon Coster, *Life* Magazine © Time Warner Inc.

150 (top) J.R. Mayall, The Francis A. Countway Library of Medicine, Harvard University

150-151 Photographer unknown, Fratelli Alinari

152 (top) Photographer unknown, © Keystone

152 (bottom) Photographer unknown, Archives, The Hospital for Sick Children, Toronto

152-153 Photographer unknown, Fratelli Alinari

154 (top) Charles O'Rear, © Westlight

154-155 Photographer unknown, St. Paul Pioneer Press

156 Photographer unknown, © Roger Viollet

157 Wilhelm Konrad Roentgen, Bettmann Archive

158-159, 159 (top) Photographer unknown, Fratelli Alinari

160-163 Alexander Tsiaras

164-165 Lennart Nilsson, © *A Child is Born,* Dell

Publishing Company

166-167 Howard Sochurek

169 Philippe Plailly, © Photo Researchers

170 Lennart Nilsson, © *A Child is Born,* Dell Publishing Company

171 Creative Media Concepts, © Boehringer Ingelheim Pharmaceuticals, Inc.

173 Seth M. Arlow, Evergreen Hospital, Kirkland, Washington

174 Nancy Leegard, Courtesy of Hennepin County Medical Center

175 Mary Pencheff, Courtesy of St. Vincent Medical Center

176 John R. Shupe, Courtesy of Primary Children's Medical Center, Salt Lake City

177 Karen Hensley, © The Methodist Hospital System, Houston

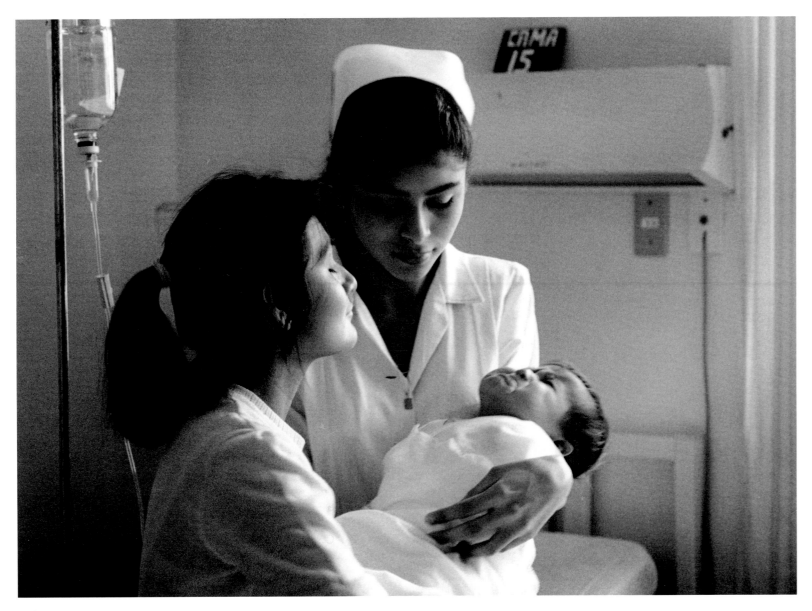

100 YEARS OF MEDICINE
PHOTO CONTEST

The *100 Years of Medicine Photo Contest* was sponsored by Olympus Camera and Hippocrates Partners, publisher of *Health* and *Hippocrates* magazines. Photo Perspectives organized the contest and issued a call for the most interesting photographs from the world of medicine and healing. The contest elicited an overwhelming response from the medical community, with hundreds of images submitted by more than two hundred health care professionals, hospital archivists, and medical photographers from across the United States and Canada. We were happily surprised to discover such a large and sophisticated community of photographers within the larger medical community. Not only was great care taken in the selection of pictures, but meticulous attention to printing, captioning, and presentation characterized many of the photographs entered. Whether depicting a makeshift dental clinic in the jungle of Guatemala, a 1912 psychiatric ward in Utah, or the frenzied effort to save lives in an Orange County emergency room, taken together the contest entries showed the strength and value of the still image in preserving in time the humanity and dedication of those individuals who are the heart of the medical community.

In connection with the *100 Years of Medicine Photo Contest* we would like to thank the following: Lauren Barnett, Director, American Society for Health Care Marketing and Public Relations, American Hospital Association; Pamela Carroll, *ACP Observer,* American College of Physicians; Herbert Gant, Director, *Psychiatric News,* American Psychiatric Association; Suzanne H. Howard, Editor, *Cardiology,* American College of Cardiologists; Judy Jakush, Editor, *ADA News,* American Dental Association; Paula S. Katz, Managing Editor, *ACP Observer,* American College of Physicians; Linn Meyer, Director of Communications, American College of Surgeons; Stephen J. Regnier, Editor, *Bulletin,* American College of Surgeons; Ronni Scheier, Assistant Executive Editor, *American Medical News,* American Medical Association; Shirley Austin, Associate Editor, *Nurseweek;* Kimburly Varnish, News and Information, *ACP Observer,* American College of Physicians; and Martha Snyder Taggart, Editor, *ACOG Newsletter.*

The *100 Years of Medicine* was judged by:
Catherine Chermayeff, Director of Special Projects, Magnum Photos and former photo editor, *Fortune;* Karen Mullarkey, former photo editor, *Newsweek, Rolling Stone,* and *Sports Illustrated;* Nan Richardson, former editor, *Aperture,* photography critic and book editor; Aaron Schindler, director, Photo Perspectives; Thomas K. Walker, GRAF/*x,* former art director, *Day in the Life* book series.

First Place Archival: Circa 1884. Alfred Harrison Neal or "Doc Neal," an Ozark physician. Photographer unknown. Submitted by his descendant Michael Duff, M.D., of Rolla, Missouri (see page 47).

Second Place Archival: Circa 1936. Grand Rounds on Skull Fracture, by Dr. George Heuer, The New York Hospital-Cornell Medical Center. Photographer unknown. Submitted by I. Michael Leitman, M.D., North Shore University Hospital (see page 67).

Third Place Archival: 1913. The first electrocardiogram performed in Chicago at Presbyterian Hospital by Lynn McBride, M.D. Photographer unknown. Submitted by Stuart Campbell, Rush-Presbyterian-St. Luke's Medical Center, Chicago, Illinois (see page 147).

Honorable Mentions Archival:
1905. State-of-the-art operation room, St. Joseph's Hospital, Parkersburg, West Virginia. Photographer unknown. Submitted by St. Joseph's Hospital.

1905. Spohn Sanatorium in Texas, where a record three hundred twenty-eight pound ovarian tumor, the largest ever, was removed from a young woman. Photographer unknown. Submitted by Aric N. Hooverson, Spohn Hospital, Corpus Christi.

1898. Newton-Wellesley Hospital School of Nursing graduation, photographer unknown. Submitted by Elizabeth J. Nedich, Newton-Wellesley Hospital, Newton, Massachusetts.

1913. Medical Students, Yale University School of Medicine. Photographer unknown. Submitted by Katherine Krauss, Yale-New Haven Hospital, New Haven, Connecticut.

1913. Operating Room. Photographer unknown. Submitted by Heidi Grim, Union Hospital, Terre Haute, Indiana.

First Place Contemporary: 1991. The Plastic Surgery Team from The Methodist Hospital in Houston's Texas Medical Center provide *pro bono* care in Chetumal, Mexico. Photographed by Karen M. Hensley (see page 177).

Second Place Contemporary: Circa 1960. The uniform and technology may change, but caring nurses are still crucial to patient care. Photographer unknown. Submitted by Nancy Leegard, Hennepin County Medical Center, Minneapolis (see page 174).

Third Place Contemporary: 1990. Pomona Valley Hospital Emergency Department. Paramedics along with fireman rush into the emergency room with patient in respiratory distress. Photographed by Elsburgh Clarke, M.D., Orange, California (see page 82).

Honorable Mentions Contemporary:
1989. Life Flight Team at scene of the auto accident. Photographed by Mary Penchoff, St. Vincent Medical Center, Toledo, Ohio (see page 175).

1991. A nurse administers to Sami Samhouri, age two. Primary Care Children's Medical Center, Salt Lake City, Utah. Photographed by John R. Shupe, Ogden, Utah (see page 176).

1990. Obstetrician performing a C-section. Photographed by John F. Smith, M.D., Submitted by Waterbury Hospital, Waterbury, Connecticut.

1989. Hip replacement operation. Photographed by Seth M. Arlow, M.D., Evergreen Hospital Medical Center, Kirkland, Washington (see page 173).

1990. Pomona Valley Hospital Emergency Department. Pomona police accompany a violent PCP suspect for medical treatment before bringing him to jail. Photographed by Elsburgh Clarke, M.D., Orange, California.